Dear DIABETES ADVISOR

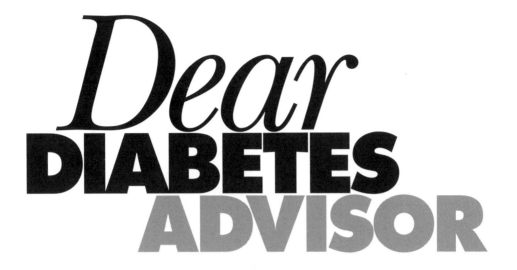

Dear DIABETES ADVISOR

Plain and Simple

Answers to

Your Questions

About Diabetes

Foreword by
Michael A. Pfeifer,
MD, MS, CDE, FACE

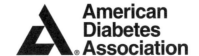
American Diabetes Association

CONTRIBUTORS
Shauna Roberts, PhD, science and health writer; Michael A. Pfeifer, MD, MS, CDE, FACE, editor of *The Diabetes Advisor* newsletter; Peter Banks, editorial director of the publications division at the American Diabetes Association; Karen Lombardi Ingle, book editor for the American Diabetes Association; Long-Run Publications, specializing in editing and production of books, magazines, manuals, and journals

BOOK EDITOR
Karen Lombardi Ingle

PRODUCTION COORDINATOR
Peggy M. Rote

PRODUCTION MANAGER
Carolyn R. Segree

BOOK DESIGN
Wickham & Associates, Inc.

TYPESETTING
Harlowe Typography, Inc.

ILLUSTRATOR
Richard Thompson

Library of Congress Cataloging-in-Publication Data

Dear diabetes advisor / foreword by Michael A. Pfeifer.
    p. cm.
    Includes index.
    ISBN 0-945448-83-X (pbk.)
    1. Diabetes—Popular works.   2. Diabetes—Miscellanea.
I. American Diabetes Association.
RC660.4.D43   1997
799.1'24—dc21
                                                                               97-10397
                                                                                 CIP

The suggestions and information contained in this publication are generally consistent with the *Clinical Practice Recommendations* and other policies of the American Diabetes Association, but they do not represent the policy or position of the Association or any of its boards or committees. Reasonable steps have been taken to ensure the accuracy of the information presented. However, the American Diabetes Association cannot ensure the safety or efficacy of any product or service described in this publication. Individuals are advised to consult a physician or other appropriate health care professional before undertaking any diet or exercise program or taking any medication referred to in this publication. Professionals must use and apply their own professional judgment, experience, and training and should not rely solely on the information contained in this publication before prescribing any diet, exercise, or medication. The American Diabetes Association—its officers, directors, employees, volunteers, and members—assumes no responsibility or liability for personal or other injury, loss, or damage that may result from the suggestions or information in this publication.

©1997 by the American Diabetes Association, Inc. All Rights Reserved. No part of this publication may be reproduced or transmitted in any form or by any means, electronic or mechanical, including duplication, recording, or any information storage and retrieval system, without the prior written permission of the American Diabetes Association.
Printed in the United States of America

American Diabetes Association
1660 Duke Street
Alexandria, Virginia 22314

American Diabetes Association
Books Editorial Advisory Board

EDITOR-IN-CHIEF

David B. Kelley, MD
  Olympia, Washington

ASSOCIATE EDITORS

Robert M. Anderson, EdD
  Michigan Diabetes Research and Training Center
  The University of Michigan Medical School
  Ann Arbor, Michigan

Janine C. Freeman, RD, CDE
  Georgia Center for Diabetes at Columbia
  Dunwoody Medical Center
  Atlanta, Georgia

Patti Bazel Geil, MS, RD, CDE
  The University of Kentucky Hospital
  Lexington, Kentucky

Marvin E. Levin, MD
  Chesterfield, Missouri

Barbara J. Maschak-Carey, RNCS, MSN, CDE
  Hospital of the University of Pennsylvania
  Philadelphia, Pennsylvania

David S. Schade, MD
  The University of New Mexico School of Medicine
  Albuquerque, New Mexico

MEMBERS

Samuel L. Abbate, MD, CDE
  Medcenter One Health Systems
  Bismarck, North Dakota

Eva Brzezinski, RD, MS
  University of California San Diego Medical Center
  General Clinical Research Center
  San Diego, California

Connie C. Crawley, RD, BS, MS
  The University of Georgia Cooperative Extension Service
  Athens, Georgia

John T. Devlin, MD
  Maine Medical Center
  Portland, Maine

Alan M. Jacobson, MD
  Joslin Diabetes Center
  Boston, Massachusetts

Lois Jovanovic, MD
  Sansum Medical Research Foundation
  Santa Barbara, California

Carolyn Leontos, MS, RD, CDE
  The University of Nevada Cooperative Extension
  Las Vegas, Nevada

Peter A. Lodewick, MD
  Diabetes Care Center
  Birmingham, Alabama

Carol E. Malcom, BSN, CDE
  Highline Community Hospital
  Seattle, Washington

Wylie McNabb, EdD
  The University of Chicago Center for Medical Education and Health Care
  Chicago, Illinois

Virginia Peragallo-Dittko, RN, MA, CDE
  Winthrop University Hospital
  Mineola, New York

Jacqueline Siegel, RN
  St. Joseph Hospital
  Seattle, Washington

Tim Wysocki, PhD
  Nemours Children's Clinic
  Jacksonville, Florida

Contents

FOREWORD ix

ACKNOWLEDGMENTS . . . xiii

Chapter 1
TREATMENT 1

Chapter 2
EXERCISE 21

Chapter 3
COPING 33

Chapter 4
**HEALTHY COOKING
AND EATING** 43

Chapter 5
WEIGHT LOSS 61

Chapter 6
INSURANCE 69

Chapter 7
CONSUMER ISSUES 83

INDEX 89

Foreword

It's April. The sun is shining brightly in my office as I sit down to pen this foreword. I have contemplated many subjects in deciding what to write. As I ponder the various topics, I hear the shrill cry of the geese as they fly across the sky, and their shadow briefly dances across my office. The shadow seems to lead to several orchids that reside in my office. My thoughts drift. I have noticed over the years that most of my orchids proliferate and prosper, while others seem to wither and die in spite of my best care. Why is this? Is there something missing? I have tried various nutrients; I have read books on the care and arrangement of orchids; I have sought consults; I have talked to the orchids and played music for them; and yet, some of these plants never seem to prosper. Some of the orchid consultants have told me I should just toss those struggling plants and begin anew. "With so many orchids," they say, "why waste your time?" "But don't these plants deserve my time and the very best of care?" I ask.

There must be a missing element. I just haven't discovered it yet. Occasionally I am able to find the problem, correct it, and get the struggling plants to bloom. Their blossoms are especially beautiful to me. Unfortunately, people with diabetes can be similar to my struggling orchids. In spite of the best care, some people are unable to avoid or delay the complications of diabetes. It is my contention that a missing element keeps these patients from avoiding these problems. The missing element is patient education. Patient education is the reason some people with diabetes are able to avoid or delay diabetes complications and have a better quality of life than others. Like my struggling orchids that bloom, these patients are especially "beautiful" to health care providers.

Of course, patient education is not the only missing element; there are certainly others. However, it is an attainable element of diabetes care. In spite of health care providers' doggedly tenacious efforts to inform patients, sometimes it's not enough. Truly appropriate care requires patients to self-manage their own diabetes. Diabetes is the only disease in which I actively encourage my patients to do their own lab testing, make diagnostic and therapeutic decisions based on the testing results, and modify their treatment regimen appropriately. Diabetes requires decision making. In order to make these decisions, people with diabetes need to be educated and informed about diabetes and its management. It is the responsibility of people with diabetes to seek, find, and obtain that needed education and information.

We live in the Information Age. Information is available from countless sources. A popular source of information these days is the Internet. Today when I surfed the net, there were nearly a quarter of a million home pages concerning diabetes and more than a thousand diabetes chat rooms. The quantity of information is impressive, no doubt. I found all sorts of information. Some of it was good, reliable information; but some of it was not. Unfortunately, quantity does not equal quality. Judging the quality of information can be difficult. So how will you know whether the information you obtain is good? Consider the source of the information. Reputable organizations like the American Diabetes Association are the best sources of valid information. It is the mission of such organizations to provide you with the most accurate, up-to-date information available.

Being informed about one's own health is a responsibility that every patient with diabetes or any chronic disease must undertake. As you gather information and educational "nutrients," in order to ensure your best chance to blossom and not to become an individual who struggles to survive (like some of my orchids), be certain of the source of the information and be wary of sources that are not monitored for accuracy. Such sources contain misinformation, which is potentially harmful to you.

Dear Diabetes Advisor answers a series of questions that patients frequently ask. The information is reliable, accurate, and invaluable. Enjoy this book; read it in a relaxed atmosphere. Most of the letters and replies are short. This allows the book to be easily picked up and put down. However, don't put it down too long. —Michael A. Pfeifer, MD

Acknowledgments

Many thanks to the reviewers of this book:

Robert M. Anderson, EdD
Michigan Diabetes Research and Training Center
The University of Michigan Medical School
Ann Arbor, Michigan

Peggy M. Batchelor
Member of the Alexandria Hospital Diabetes Support Group

Eva Brzezinski, RD, MS
University of California San Diego Medical Center
General Clinical Research Center
San Diego, California

Bill Byrd
Member of the Alexandria Hospital Diabetes Support Group

David B. Kelley, MD
Olympia, Washington

Carol E. Malcom, BSN, CDE
Highline Community Hospital
Seattle, Washington

David S. Schade, MD
The University of New Mexico School of Medicine
Albuquerque, New Mexico

Chapter one: TREATMENT

Ouch! When I eat a big meal, I get a pain in my stomach on the right side. Is this diabetes? Or could it be my gallbladder giving out?

It may very well be your gallbladder. A gallbladder problem can cause pain. The pain may make you feel sick to your stomach. Usually, you feel the pain just under your breastbone or to its right. The pain often starts after you eat or while you are sleeping.

Stones may form in the gallbladder. Gallstones are actually more common in people with diabetes than in people without diabetes. Usually, gallstones sit quietly in the gallbladder, causing no problems. But occasionally, a stone sticks in the bile duct. The bile duct is a tube that takes bile (an aid to digestion that is made in the liver and stored in the gallbladder) to the intestines. When the bile duct is plugged, bile builds up in the gallbladder, causing swelling, inflammation, and intense pain.

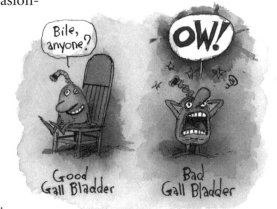

People with diabetes whose gallstones start acting up are more likely to get severe inflammation than people without diabetes. Inflammation is most likely when diabetes is in poor control.

Gallstones may be destroyed with ultrasound or dissolved with pills. But the main treatment for gallstones is an opera-

TREATMENT 1

tion to remove the gallbladder and, with it, the stones. This operation is called a cholecystectomy. After the operation, your liver will deposit bile directly into your intestines.

My dentist says people with diabetes can have a lot of dental problems. How can I protect my teeth?

Your dentist is correct. High glucose levels in blood and tissues provide a feast for bacteria. This can increase the likelihood of your developing gum disease and other mouth infections.

Fortunately, if you know what problems can happen and how to prevent them, you can keep that drill out of your dentist's hand and your teeth in your mouth. Here are some ways to keep your teeth healthy:

- Keep your blood glucose under good control. Be aware that dental problems can actually cause poor control.

- Brush at least twice a day and floss once a day. A soft toothbrush is best.

- Have your teeth cleaned by a dentist or dental hygienist every 6 months.

- Make sure your dentist takes full mouth X rays every 2 years to check for bone loss. Some people have no external symptoms of gum disease.

- Know the warning signs of gum problems: gums that bleed when you brush or floss, red or swollen gums, gums that have pulled away from your teeth, pus in your gums, bad breath, loose teeth, shifting teeth, and dentures that no longer fit well.

- Know the warning signs of infections. Bacterial or fungal infections may cause swelling, pus, white or red patches, pain, or dark spots on your teeth. Your teeth may become sensitive to temperature changes or sweets.

My doctor has put me on insulin and diabetes pills. Isn't this a bit much? Why won't one medication do?

Picture Batman and Robin. Yeah, each one of them might be able to fight crime on his own, but together they've got that dynamic duo thing going. It's the same with diabetes pills and insulin, although it's called combination therapy.

Combining diabetes pills and insulin is not the same as taking more of one or the other, because diabetes pills and insulin work in different ways. People with type 2 diabetes have two problems. The first problem is that their bodies resist the action of insulin. Insulin's job is to help store glucose in cells. So insulin resistance leads to glucose building up in the blood. The second problem is that the pancreas secretes too little insulin.

Insulin helps when the pancreas makes too little insulin. Some diabetes pills affect the level of insulin: sulfonylureas help your body make more of its own insulin, while thiazolidinediones enhance the action of insulin so that your body needs less. Other diabetes pills affect the level of glucose: biguanides slow the release of stored glucose from your liver, while alpha-glucosidase inhibitors slow the time it takes your intestine to break down starches and certain sugars into glucose. Because of these different effects, pills and insulin together may help you more than either alone.

With combination therapy, you may be able to take less insulin or get smoother blood glucose control. Your doctor can tell you specifically why one medication alone didn't work as well for you.

I feel like a medical specimen. Not only do I have diabetes but also high blood pressure and arthritis. How can I manage all these pills and doctor visits?

 People with diabetes often have diabetes plus something else. That something else could be heart disease, high blood fat (cholesterol and triglyceride) levels, or arthritis or high blood pressure. Dubbed "diabetes plus," these multiple conditions make life trickier. Besides having more doctors to deal with and more drugs to juggle, the treatment for one condition may make another one worse. Here are some ways to deal with the double trouble of diabetes plus:

- Have one doctor be in charge. Having one doctor as your team leader ensures someone is looking out for you as a whole person. It gives you someone to help you sort out the conflicting demands and to mediate between the other team members.

- Keep all your doctors informed. Don't play favorites. Tell every doctor you see that you have diabetes plus other conditions. Also, tell each what drugs you are taking. Each time a doctor prescribes a new medicine or treatment, ask how it will affect your diabetes. Ask as well whether it will interact with your other drugs and treatments.

- Go to only one pharmacy, if possible. It's time to become pals with your pharmacist. He or she will be better able to warn you of possible drug interactions if he or she knows the other drugs you take. You can also buy a book about drugs and their interactions.

- Read, read, read. Knowledge is power. Knowing about your health problems is even more vital when you have several. At the very least, you want to learn enough to know which doctor to see when something goes wrong.

- Give yourself a break. Battling more than one chronic disease at the same time is rough. Be kind to yourself, and take rest breaks if you need to. Learn to say no when others' demands are too much for you.

- Keep notes. A notebook will help you keep track of your doctors and their suggestions and treatments. Take the notebook each time you go to a doctor. If one doctor needs to know about a treatment prescribed by one of the others or needs to contact that doctor, you will have the information at hand.

- Keep a list of questions to ask. Studies have shown that people who ask questions have better health overall than people who don't.

• •

I have blocked arteries in my heart, and I'm trying to decide with my doctor what treatment is best. My doctor says bypass surgery is safer than balloon angioplasty, but I'm worried about having surgery. Do you have information on what's best?

You would think that using that little balloon thing to open up your arteries would be better, but it's not. Results from an ongoing study have found that more people with diabetes survive bypass surgery than balloon angioplasty.

Researchers have been following 1,829 people who had two or more blocked arteries. Half had bypass surgery. In bypass surgery, a healthy vein is taken from another part of the body and sewn onto the blocked artery above and below the blockage. Blood then makes a detour around the blockage.

The other patients had balloon angioplasty. In balloon angioplasty, a balloon is inserted into the artery and inflated at the blockage. The artery stretches. Blood has room to flow past the clog.

Five years after the treatments, the researchers found the death rate was twice as high after balloon angioplasty as after bypass surgery in the 353 people who took insulin or pills for diabetes. For people who did not have diabetes, both procedures were equally safe.

The National Institutes of Health now recommends that people with diabetes who take insulin or pills and who have two or more blocked arteries have bypass surgery rather than balloon angioplasty.

I don't get sick often, but my doctor says I should have a flu shot. Seems like a waste of money to me, but should I get one because of my diabetes?

Obviously you haven't had the flu lately. Let me refresh your memory: days and days of chills, fever, muscle aches, headache, sore throat, and cough. Believe me, you don't want it, so just play it safe and get the flu shot.

Each year, about 20,000 Americans die from the flu. People with diabetes are more likely to die from the flu or pneumonia than people without diabetes. Sometimes, the flu can lead to pneumonia.

Most people with diabetes are advised to get a flu shot once a year, in October. The shot makes it harder to catch the flu for about 6 months. Even if you do catch the flu, your symptoms will likely be milder than they otherwise would have been (hey, every little bit helps). It may be a good idea for your family members and roommates to have flu shots, too. Then you won't catch the flu from them.

If you are allergic to eggs, you may be allergic to the flu shot, so check with your doctor first before getting one. Also, if you have a cold, wait until you're healthy again before having your flu shot. Ask your doctor about getting a pneumonia shot as well. Many people with diabetes need one every 5 or 6 years.

My doctor says my cholesterol level is too high. Why should I care, and what do I do to lower cholesterol?

Why should you care? People with diabetes tend to have higher levels of LDL (the bad) cholesterol and lower levels of HDL (the good) cholesterol. LDL cholesterol can stick to blood vessel walls and clog arteries. A high level of LDL cholesterol in your blood puts you at risk for heart disease, heart attack, and stroke. In addition, 80 percent of people with diabetes die from a disease of the blood vessels or heart. Now do you care? I thought so. Here are some things you can do to lower your cholesterol level:

- Control your diabetes. When your diabetes is out of control, none of the other steps will help as much.
- Lose weight if you need to. Excess weight raises cholesterol levels.
- Become more physically active. Try aerobic exercises, such as brisk walking, jogging, swimming, and skiing. Exercise raises your good HDL cholesterol.
- Cut back on all the fat in your diet. Fat does more to raise your cholesterol level than anything else.
- Replace saturated fats (butter, lard) with unsaturated fats (most vegetable oils). Saturated fats raise your cholesterol level, while unsaturated fats may lower it.
- Eat high-cholesterol foods less often. Foods high in cholesterol include organ meats, such as liver, and egg yolks. If you eat eggs every day, try cutting back to three or four a week.
- Eat foods high in fiber. Some types of fiber help remove cholesterol from the body. Oats, beans, peas, fresh fruits, and brown rice are great fiber choices.
- If you smoke, cut down or quit. Quitting smoking raises your good HDL cholesterol.
- Ask your doctor about cholesterol-lowering medications.

I've just been put on acarbose, but I'm not sure why. What is the drug supposed to do?

Acarbose (brand name Precose) is a pill that slows down the time it takes for your intestine to break down starches and double sugars into glucose. (Sucrose or table sugar is a double sugar. It is made up of glucose and fructose, which are single sugars. Single sugars don't need to be broken down in the intestine. They're already small enough to be absorbed.) This delay causes glucose to enter your blood more slowly. Your blood glucose then stays more even, with fewer highs and lows. Acarbose helps flatten out the sharp rise in glucose that may occur after meals loaded with starches and double sugars.

You take acarbose with the first bite of each of your main meals. Acarbose slows the breakdown of breads, crackers, cereals, grains, and pasta; beans, potatoes, and vegetables; and white (table) sugar, brown sugar, powdered sugar, maple syrup, molasses, and beer. Acarbose has little or no effect on the breakdown of glucose tablets or gel, corn syrup, honey, fruits, milk, or yogurt.

Acarbose, by itself, doesn't cause low blood glucose reactions. But if you are also taking insulin or a sulfonylurea, your blood glucose level may drop too low on occasion. If you have a low blood glucose reaction, it is safest to treat it with something that is not affected by acarbose, such as glucose tablets or gel.

The side effects of acarbose are gas, bloating, and diarrhea. You may get these side effects when you start taking acarbose. After a time, these side effects usually go away. If you have problems with your intestines, have had abdominal surgery, or have gastroparesis, you should not take acarbose.

I've tried to talk with my doctor about neuropathy pain, and he says there's nothing to do but grin and bear it. Well, I'm not grinning. What can I do?

 First find a doctor who is more knowledgeable about painful diabetic neuropathy. While it's true that there's no drug that can cure neuropathy, there are things you can do to slow down its progress and reduce the pain.

To Slow Its Progress
- Get your blood glucose level under control.
- Quit smoking.
- Drink less alcohol.
- Keep your blood pressure under control.
- Keep your cholesterol level low.

To Reduce the Pain
- Try low-impact exercises. Exercising may be the last thing you want to do. But oddly enough, walking, swimming, and other low-impact exercises may reduce your pain. Be sure to avoid those that are hard on your feet, such as jogging.
- Protect your feet in bed. One solution is to wear heavy socks. Another is to lift the sheets off your feet. Try putting a Hula Hoop or wire rack at the end of your bed.
- Try stretching exercises if you have muscle pain. Tight muscles hurt. Stretching and massage can force the muscle to relax.
- Try over-the-counter capsaicin cream if you have skin pain. It's made from hot peppers. You may experience a burning sensation at first, but after you've used it for a couple of weeks, skin pain may lessen.
- See a doctor who has treated people with painful diabetic neuropathy. He or she will be able to prescribe a drug to relieve your specific type of pain.

- See a therapist. Sometimes, people get depressed when pain goes on and on. Getting your depression treated can help your pain.

• •

I'm a 50-year-old man who doesn't even want to think about prostate problems. Still, I know I should. What do I really need to know?

You are right to be worried about your prostate. As men grow older, their prostates may grow and cause problems. Benign prostatic hyperplasia (BPH) is the most common medical problem of men over age 55. BPH means that the prostate has gotten bigger but does not contain cancer. This growth compresses the urethra (the tube through which urine passes), making it difficult or uncomfortable (burning or stinging) to urinate. You may need to urinate more often, perhaps getting up several times a night. If you have these symptoms, go see a doctor.

BPH treatment options include finasteride, a drug that shrinks the prostate; terazosin or doxazosin, drugs that relax bladder and prostate muscles; and removal or destruction of the prostate by surgery, laser, heat, microwaves, or vaporization.

Now for the even more scary stuff. Prostate cancer is the most common cancer men get. About 9 percent of older men develop prostate cancer. The older you are, the slower prostate cancer is likely to grow. Men with slow-growing cancers may live a full life span without treatment. Because prostate cancer is so common, every man (and that includes you) needs to take certain steps.

The American Cancer Society (ACS) suggests that you have a digital rectal exam every year after you're 40 (quit whimpering, it's not that bad). ACS also suggests having a prostate-specific antigen blood test yearly after you're 50.

Treatment options for prostate cancer include surgically removing the prostate; killing tumor cells with radiation or freezing; lowering male sex hormone levels, which spur prostate growth, by castration or hormone treatment; and "watching and waiting," which means having regular checkups but not taking any drastic actions unless the tumor starts growing faster. Discuss these treatment options in depth with your doctor. Every treatment has both good and bad points.

Everybody says to insist on good diabetes care. But, what is good diabetes care, and how do I make sure I'm getting it?

To help you determine whether you are getting good care, the American Diabetes Association has developed "Standards of Medical Care for Patients with Diabetes Mellitus" (published each year in Supplement 1 of the January issue of *Diabetes Care*). This report tells your health care team how to take care of you. For example, at your initial visit, your health care team should

- Ask when you found out you had diabetes
- Ask for results of those lab tests
- Ask who else in your family has diabetes
- Ask how you treat your diabetes
- Ask what and when you eat
- Ask how often and how hard you exercise
- Ask about your weight
- Ask if you smoke, have high blood pressure, or have high cholesterol
- Ask if you have had low blood glucose reactions or ketones in your urine
- Ask what infections or complications you have had
- Ask what treatments you have been given
- Ask what drugs you are taking
- Ask what other medical problems you have had
- Measure your height, weight, and blood pressure

- Look in your eyes and ask about eye problems
- Look in your mouth and ask about dental problems
- Feel your neck to check your thyroid gland, and do tests if needed
- Listen to your heart through a stethoscope, and take your pulse
- Feel your abdomen to check your liver and other organs
- Look at your hands and fingers
- Look at your bare feet, and check the sensation and pulses in your feet
- Check your skin
- Request blood and urine samples for tests
- Provide you with a diabetes management plan

Your diabetes management plan should include

- A list of goals
- A list of the medications that you use for diabetes
- A plan for healthy eating
- A list of lifestyle changes for you to make, such as getting more exercise
- Education in diabetes self-management
- Training on how to self-monitor your blood glucose, test your urine for ketones, and keep records
- A plan for caring for your teeth, your feet, your skin
- A plan for sick days and pregnancy
- Referral to specialists, such as an eye doctor and a foot doctor, as needed
- Instructions on when to come back and when to call

I'm going on 80, and I just got diabetes. My doctor says to take care of it, but I'm too old to learn new things. Any hints for this old dog?

Just because you're getting on in years does not mean that dealing with diabetes will be extra hard. In fact, the skills and wisdom you've acquired in your journey through life may help you deal with diabetes better than younger folks.

Although you may not be as mentally spry as you once were, you can improve your brain power. Regular exercise sends extra oxygen to the brain and may help you think faster. Mental challenges—from working crossword puzzles and brain teasers to taking college classes or dancing lessons—may also help keep you sharp.

Also, keep in mind your big advantage over young 'uns—you've been through many troubles in your life and seen amazing changes in society. So you already have lots of experience adapting to changes.

And don't forget that you still have plenty of years left to enjoy if you take care of yourself. Good diabetes control does not just have benefits down the road. It will also help you have more energy and feel better now.

Another motivating factor for taking care of your diabetes is the effect you have on other people. Without trying to sound too melodramatic, you're never too old to make a difference in the world. Not only will your children and grandchildren miss you if you die too early, but so will all the other people you might have helped or inspired. End of sermon. Now start learning some new tricks.

I'm a woman in my early 30s, and I want to do all I can to avoid the kind of osteoporosis that my mother has. What steps can I take now to protect myself later in life?

The fact that you're starting at a relatively young age already gives you a better chance of preventing osteoporosis. There are several things you can do to protect your bones.

- See your doctor to be evaluated for early signs of osteoporosis, especially if you have risk factors, such as being small-boned, white or Asian, or inactive. Certain medications may slow the progress of osteoporosis.

- Eat a diet rich in calcium. The RDA (Recommended Dietary Allowance) for calcium for men and women in your age group (age 25 and above) is 800 mg per day. Some low-fat sources of this mineral include skim milk, low-fat or nonfat yogurt, low-fat or nonfat cheeses, greens (collards, turnip greens, mustard greens, etc.), broccoli, spinach, peas and beans, and low-fat tofu.

- If you are lactose intolerant, consider taking a calcium supplement.

- Do weight-bearing exercises, such as lifting weights, running, and hiking. Weight-bearing exercises stimulate the body to add more bone.

- Take extra calcium when you are pregnant. The RDA for calcium when you are pregnant is 1,200 mg a day.

- When you get past menopause, talk to your doctor about taking estrogen. Estrogen can slow bone loss.

- Get the men in your life into the act, too. Men are not immune to osteoporosis. In fact, more than 2 million American men have osteoporosis.

I'm a 39-year-old man having trouble with my sex life. Are treatments available?

I'm going to assume that the trouble you are referring to is impotence. Impotence occurs 3 times as often in men with diabetes as in those without diabetes at the same age. Treatments for impotence depend on the cause. A doctor can help identify the cause of your impotence. Psychological, drug-related, hormonal, and blood flow-related causes of impotence all have specific treatments. Impotence caused by trauma, surgery (especially prostate surgery), or nerve damage to the penis is treated similarly.

One treatment for these latter causes of impotence is to inject a drug, such as papaverine, phentolamine, or alprostadil, into the side of the penis. These drugs cause an erection that lasts about 30 minutes to an hour. Another method requires you to insert a pellet of a drug (such as alprostadil) into your urethra (the tube through which urine passes). In another method, you take a pill by mouth (not FDA-approved at this writing). Other treatments for impotence include using a vacuum pump to create an erection and surgically implanting prosthetic devices in the penis.

I have so many darn medicines to take I get confused. How can I keep all this straight, short of having a nurse follow me around?

It's worth it to put some time and effort into getting your medicines straight. Here are some hints for mastering the mysteries of medicine taking:

- Take your medicines on time each day. If the label says something vague like "4 times a day" or "3 times a day," ask your doctor or pharmacist specifically when to take it.

- Get a pill box or tray with enough compartments in it for the day or week. You can label it by time of day or event, such as "before breakfast." You may want to keep at least one pill in the original bottle at home in case you forget which pill is which.

- Make a daily chart for your medicines. If you check off each drug as you swallow it, you won't lose track of whether you've taken it yet.

- Some medicines should be taken with food; others should be taken on an empty stomach. Know which of yours are which.

- Turn on the light before taking a medicine at night.

- Be sure you know where and how to take or apply the medicine.

- Make sure you've poured the right dose before swallowing. It's easy to mix up the lines marking teaspoons and tablespoons, for example.

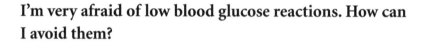

I'm very afraid of low blood glucose reactions. How can I avoid them?

Low blood glucose reactions, also known as hypoglycemia, are certainly scary and can be dangerous. You may get low blood glucose if you use insulin or take sulfonylureas (a class of diabetes pills). Low blood glucose reactions are more common if you are trying to get your blood glucose level as close to normal as possible (known as tight control). Here are some tips that may help you avoid low blood glucose reactions:

- Eat meals and snacks on time. Don't skip any.
- Be sure to eat enough food.
- Be careful not to overexercise.
- Be careful not to get dehydrated.
- Take the right amount of insulin or number of diabetes pills.
- Test your glucose more often, especially when you are sick.
- Don't drink alcohol on an empty stomach.

Treat Low Blood Glucose With One of These Foods

Glucose tablets or gel (the dose is printed on the package)
1/2 cup (4 ounces) of fruit juice
1/3 can (4 ounces) of a regular (not diet) soft drink
1 cup (8 ounces) of skim milk
1 tablespoon of honey or syrup
2 tablespoons of raisins (40–50)
3 graham crackers
4 teaspoons of granulated sugar
6 saltine crackers
6 1/2-inch sugar cubes

Ask your health care team for the treatment options that are best for you.

- Talk to your health care team about trying a different insulin regimen. Changing the timing of your shots, where you inject them, or the type of insulin might suit your body better.
- Consider an insulin pump. Pumps imitate the natural release of insulin better than shots do.
- Get to know your own warning signs of low blood glucose. They may be different from those someone else feels. Tell your signs to someone who can help you watch out for them.
- Participate in blood glucose awareness training, if possible. These classes teach you to cue in to your body so that you can recognize low blood glucose levels early.
- When any of your warning signs occur, treat low blood glucose right away. Always, always have something on hand for treating reactions.

I'm a 25-year-old woman with diabetes who'd like to have a baby. What do I need to do before I get pregnant?

Most women with diabetes can have a safe and successful pregnancy. Here's what you need to do:

- Get your blood glucose in good control (i.e., between 70 and 100 mg/dl before meals; less than 140 mg/dl at 1 hour after meals; and less than 120 mg/dl at 2 hours after meals). If your blood glucose is in poor control, try to bring it into good control 3 to 6 months before you plan to get pregnant. If you wait until you know you are pregnant, your baby could already be harmed. High blood glucose levels during the first 8 weeks of your pregnancy can cause birth defects. It is during these early weeks that your baby's organs are forming.

- Get fit. Exercising before pregnancy may increase your endurance, help lower your blood glucose, help you lose weight, and build strength and flexibility.

- Avoid drinking alcohol, smoking cigarettes, and using illegal drugs. All of these can harm your baby.

- If you have any diabetes complications, consult your doctor about whether pregnancy could worsen your complication.

- If you have a gynecological problem that could make it harder for you to get pregnant or stay pregnant, you may want to have it fixed now.

   Your health care team will set up a pregnancy plan for you. It will include a meal plan, an exercise plan, and a schedule for insulin and self-monitoring of blood glucose.

Ever since I got diabetes, my skin has been dry and itchy. What can I do for relief?

Try the following tips for your dry and itchy skin:

- Keep your diabetes in good control. High blood glucose levels can lead to damaged sweat glands over time, which can leave you with dry skin.
- Take warm, not hot, baths or showers. Hot water can dry out your skin.
- Dry off right away instead of letting water evaporate and dry out your skin.
- Use moisturizers and moisturizing soaps. Avoid products in which an alcohol is one of the first three ingredients. Words that end in "-ol" are usually alcohols. Alcohol can dry your skin even more.
- Keep your home more humid during cold, dry months.
- Drink plenty of water. It helps keep your skin moist, too.
- Protect your skin from the sun. The sun can dry and burn your skin. When you are out in the sun, wear a waterproof, sweatproof sunscreen with an SPF (sun protection factor) of at least 15. Wearing clothing and a hat also helps.
- See a skin doctor (dermatologist). If you are prone to skin problems, ask your diabetes care doctor about adding a skin doctor to your health care team.

Chapter two: EXERCISE

I exercise a lot. All my exercise partners take along sports drinks, but the first ingredient of these drinks is sugar. Are they safe for me to use?

Yes, they are safe, so feel free to join the crowd. If you are exercising for 60 minutes or longer, a sports drink can be useful. The carbohydrates in it can give you an energy boost. Also, a sports drink can help keep your blood glucose level from falling too low if you take insulin or sulfonylureas (a class of diabetes pills).

Another option is to drink diluted fruit juice (a mixture of half juice and half water). Diluted fruit juice is absorbed as quickly as a sports drink (full-strength fruit juice is absorbed more slowly) and will also keep your blood glucose level from going too low during long or hard exercising.

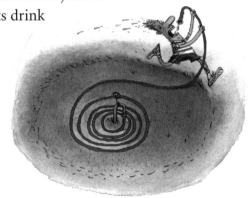

If you are exercising for less than 60 minutes, cool water is probably the best fluid to drink. Avoid alcohol and soft drinks with caffeine. These can dehydrate you. Also, carbonated beverages can make you feel fuller, causing you to not drink enough.

It's important to drink enough fluids before and after exercise and, if the exercise is intense, during exercise. Check your blood glucose level before and every 30 minutes during exercise. If your blood glucose level is stable, and you don't want or need the sugar in a regular sports drink, you might try one of the "light" sports drinks. Gatorade Light is sweetened with saccharin and has half the carbohydrates of regular Gatorade.

"No pain, no gain," my coaches used to tell me. But I've got enough aches and pains without looking for more from exercise. Is there a pain-free way to gain?

I can tell you that one of the biggest myths about exercising is that if it doesn't hurt, it's not working. Pain during exercise may be caused by any number of things. You may have poor circulation in your legs, for example. Maybe the exercise is not safe for you (see footnote).

Maybe you are not doing the exercise the right way. If you do exercises the wrong way, you can injure yourself. If you are not certain about the way to do an exercise, ask someone who does know, such as a physical therapist, an exercise physiologist, or a fitness instructor.

Maybe you did not warm up enough. Each time you exercise, it is important to warm up for 5 to 10 minutes before the exercise and cool down for 5 to 10 minutes after the exercise. A warm-up will slowly raise your heart rate, warm your muscles, and help prevent injuries. A cooldown will lower your heart rate and slow your breathing. As a warm-up or a cooldown, you could slowly walk or slowly bicycle, then gently stretch.

Maybe you are trying to do too much too soon. If you are just starting to exercise after a long time of little or no activity, go slowly. Doing too much too fast or doing more than you are capable of can lead to painful injuries.

Start with just 5 minutes of aerobic exercise each day for 1 or 2 weeks. Add 5 more minutes, then another 5. Gradually build up to doing 20 to 60 minutes of continuous aerobic exercise 3 to 5 times a week.

You can even try spreading out your exercise over the day. For example, you might try brisk walking or stair climbing for

10 minutes 2 or 3 times a day or for 15 minutes twice a day. Hopefully, you'll find this invigorating and not painful.

Check with your doctor before starting any exercise program. Some exercises may not be safe for your eyes, feet, kidneys, heart, or blood pressure.

Exercise and I don't mix. But I might be able to walk a little more than I do now. How do I start?

Ah, the old oil and vinegar excuse, "Exercise and I don't mix." Well, if you shake up oil and vinegar they do mix long enough for you to enjoy your salad. So I'm going to shake you up by scrambling some of the most common excuses for not starting a walking program.

- "I have nowhere to walk." If your neighborhood is not safe, try walking in a mall. You may also be able to walk near your office before work or over your lunch break. You could join the zoo or botanical gardens so that you get in for free and can go as often as you like.

- "I can't afford a bunch of costly equipment just for exercising." You don't need fancy clothes or devices to walk. The one piece of equipment you do need is a good pair of walking shoes.

- "I don't have time to walk." You can do it in bits and pieces. Walk to lunch instead of driving. Park at the far end of the parking lot. Get off the bus a block or two early. Don't call co-workers with questions, walk to their desks.

- "I don't know how to do it right." Hey, you've been walking since you were a baby. If you want a harder workout, just swing your arms and walk a bit faster.

- "I don't want to walk by myself." Ask friends, relatives, or neighbors whether they would enjoy walking with you. If not, join a mall-walking club.

EXERCISE 23

- "Walking hurts." You may feel sharp pains in your calves when you walk (intermittent claudication). This pain is caused by poor circulation. Walking is one of the best treatments for this condition. You may have a compressed nerve in your foot (tarsal tunnel syndrome). Special prescription shoes can protect and cushion your feet. Heavily padded socks can also help. Your muscles may become sore if you are trying to do too much too soon. Try walking less far or less fast at first. Be sure to warm up and stretch your muscles before walking.

Hopefully, I've shaken you up enough so that you and exercise do mix. Now get out there and do it. Make exercise a part of your day.

Check with your doctor before starting any exercise program. Some exercises may not be safe for your eyes, feet, kidneys, heart, or blood pressure.

I'm starting to walk a lot, but the podiatrist says to wear good shoes. How do I choose good walking shoes?

Diabetes can be a blessing in disguise when it comes to shoes. Finally, women have a good excuse to stop wearing those tight, tortuous high-heeled toe squishers, and men can stop wearing those cowboy boots with heels and pointy toes. Slip on a comfortable, well-fitting pair of walking shoes instead—what a relief, what a pleasure. Here are tips for selecting the right shoe:

- Go to the shoe store at the end of the day. That's when your feet are most swollen.
- Have a fitter measure your feet for length and width. Do it even if you've had it done recently.
- Buy by fit, not by size. You may need a larger or smaller size than usual in some styles or brands.
- Feel inside the shoe. Make sure everything is smooth. What seems like a tiny seam now could cause a blister after your foot rubs against it for hours.

- If you normally wear padded or bulky socks, wear them when you try on the shoes.

- Make sure your toes are not bunched up in the shoe (if you want that, stick with high heels and cowboy boots). About half an inch of space between the end of your toes and the shoe is good.

- Walk around. *Pay attention to any tightness or chafing.* Does the shoe rub at your ankle? *Pay attention to fit.* Does your heel rise out of the shoe? *Pay attention to how heavy they feel.* Does the shoe make you feel like you're lugging around weights? *Pay attention to the padding.* Does the shoe have enough cushioning so that you don't feel pebbles? Could you stand or walk in them for many hours? *Pay attention to shock absorption.* Does the shoe absorb the jolt when your heel hits the pavement with the weight of your whole body on it? *Pay attention to support.* Does the shoe provide enough rigidity to keep your foot from rolling or twisting?

- If you have nerve damage in your feet, then it may be harder for you to feel how the shoe fits. Bring a friend along with you to watch your heels and feet as you walk in the shoe.

- Can't bear the thought of wearing sneakers to the office? Consider dressy walking shoes. While they may not offer as much support or padding as a true walking shoe, they can be more comfortable and supportive than a dress shoe designed with only fashion in mind.

• •

I've lost just enough weight to see my toes. Now I'd like to touch them. Any hints on getting an old body more flexible?

Congratulations on losing weight. As you think about becoming more flexible, you probably remember how, when you were young, you could bend every which way at the drop of a hat. But not now.

EXERCISE 25

One of the best ways to become more flexible is to stretch every day. There are lots of different stretches. You can find them in books, on videos, and in exercise classes. Here are a few stretches for you to try. But first, some rules:

- Go slowly and smoothly.
- Remember to breathe.
- Don't bounce.
- Relax any tension you feel.
- Go only as far as you can without pain.
- Hold for at least 8 to 10 seconds.

Neck stretch. Center your head over your shoulders. Look down and let your head roll toward your chest. Bring your head back to the center. Look up and point your chin at the ceiling. Return to the center. Look over one shoulder. Return to the center. Look over the other shoulder. Return to the center. Repeat.

Arms stretch. Raise your arms over your head. Lace your fingers together with palms up. Press your arms upward. Release and lower. Repeat.

Shoulders and chest stretch. Lace your fingers together behind you. Lift your arms up. Release and lower. Repeat.

Calf stretch. Face a wall, about a foot away. Stand with one foot in front of the other, toes straight ahead. Keep both feet flat on the floor. Bend your front knee. Lean forward and rest your forearms on the wall. Press your rear heel into the floor. Repeat with other leg.

Quadriceps (front of thigh) stretch. Stand with legs straight or slightly bent. Bend one leg back, lifting your foot off the floor. Grab the ankle of the bent leg with one hand. You may need to hold on to something for balance. Gently pull your foot up so your heel is headed for your bottom and hold. Release. Repeat with other leg.

Hamstrings (back of thigh) stretch. Lie on your back. Bend your legs, feet on the floor. Lift one leg up. Keep it slightly bent.

Grasp the leg at the calf with both hands. Holding on to your leg, try to straighten it. Release. Straighten again and release. Repeat with other leg.

Lower back stretch. Lie on your back. Bring your knees to your chest. Hug your knees to your chest with your arms and press your lower back into the floor. Release arms. Lower legs.

If you would like more of a challenge, consider taking a class in a flexibility exercise like tai chi or yoga. Always watch at least one class before signing up. Also, ask whether the teacher has experience teaching students with diabetes.

Check with your doctor before starting any exercise program. Some exercises may not be safe for your eyes, feet, kidneys, heart, or blood pressure.

• •

I've never liked the way I look, and I'd like to start a weight-training program. What are the basics?

You have chosen a good time to start lifting weights. Washboard abs are in, spare tires are out. It's time to get "buff," as the young folks say.

Before you start a weight-training program, talk with your doctor or exercise physiologist to find out which exercises are safe for you (see footnote).

When you know the kinds of strength exercises that are safe for you, pick out 8 to 10 different ones. Be sure to pick ones that will work all your muscle groups: legs and hips, chest, back, shoulders, arms, and abdomen.

Once you have chosen your exercises, learn the right way to do them. If you do exercises the wrong way, you might injure yourself. If the exercises you have chosen require you to use equipment that is new to you, learn how to use and adjust it. Find out how to use any safety equipment that goes along with your exercise, too. Consider exercising with a partner (called a "spotter"). Your spotter can help you if something goes wrong.

Warm up for 5 to 10 minutes before you begin, and cool down for 5 to 10 minutes after you finish. After you warm up,

EXERCISE 27

start with just 1 set of each exercise. (A set is the number of times you repeat an exercise before you rest.) Work your way up to 2 or 3 sets of each exercise. Once you are doing 2 or 3 sets easily, then you are ready to make the exercise harder by adding more weight. Here are some general guidelines:

- To build endurance, choose a weight you can lift 15 to 20 times. Rest for 1 minute or less between sets.
- To build both strength and endurance, choose a weight you can lift 8 to 12 times. Rest for 1 or 2 minutes between sets.
- To build strength, choose a weight you can lift 2 to 6 times. Rest for 3 to 5 minutes between sets.

Move your muscles through their full range of motion. A muscle that moves only part of the way loses flexibility. And keep breathing! Breathe in as you lower. Breathe out as you lift. If you don't like this pattern, then just breathe normally.

Do strength exercises for 20 to 30 minutes 2 or 3 times a week. Allow your muscles at least 1 day of rest between days you do the same strength exercises. To grow stronger, muscles need rest as well as exercise.

Check with your doctor before starting any exercise program. Some exercises may not be safe for your eyes, feet, kidneys, heart, or blood pressure.

• •

 Let's get real. I've never exercised, and I'm not about to take up strenuous exercise now. How little could I get away with and still gain some benefit from exercise?

 Well, when it comes to exercise, I have some good news and some bad news for you. The good news is, doing any amount of exercise is better than doing none at all. The bad news is that nobody really knows the minimum amount of exercise that you can "get away with."

For the most benefit, experts recommend 20 to 30 minutes of aerobic exercise 3 or more times a week and 20 to 30 minutes of muscle strengthening and stretching exercise at least twice a week. By these guidelines, you can get away with exercising for 20 minutes a day 5 times a week—only 1 hour and 40 minutes total.

Some research has shown that exercising moderately for 15 minutes a day 3 times a week—for a total of 45 minutes—is the absolute minimum you can do and still get some health benefits. But this has not been proven conclusively. To figure out what "moderate" exercise means for you, talk with your diabetes educator. Hopefully once you start, you'll discover that exercise can be enjoyable and rewarding. Maybe you'll even want to do more.

Check with your doctor before starting any exercise program. Some exercises may not be safe for your eyes, feet, kidneys, heart, or blood pressure.

• •

I hate exercise, but I love to dance. Does dancing count as exercise?

Was Fred Astaire fat and flabby? Was Gene Kelly a couch potato? Heck no. That's because dancing is a great way to stay in shape. It's an aerobic exercise. Aerobic exercises are ones that use your heart, lungs, arms, and legs. By working these parts of your body, dancing, like all aerobic exercises, can

- Improve circulation
- Lower blood pressure
- Lower LDL cholesterol and triglycerides
- Raise HDL cholesterol (the good kind)
- Reduce body fat
- Build endurance
- Tone and strengthen muscles
- Improve flexibility and coordination
- Improve posture
- Improve the way insulin works in the body

EXERCISE 29

Get out on the dance floor for 20 minutes of continuous vigorous dancing 3 times a week, and you'll be well on your way to better health. Vigorous dancing can burn 250 calories or more per hour. Another benefit is that overuse injuries are unlikely, because you are constantly moving and changing position.

I don't know what your favorite type of dancing is, but since you love it so much you might want to try others, such as ballroom dancing, nightclub dancing, square dancing, country-western dancing, Cajun dancing, folk dancing, ballet, tap, modern dance, and jazz. Happy steppin'!

Check with your doctor before starting any exercise program. Some exercises may not be safe for your eyes, feet, kidneys, heart, or blood pressure.

 I have arthritis, so running is out for me. Still, I'd like to move around a bit. What can you tell me about pool exercises?

 Being in water is a little like being in space. You can float and move as if you weighed very little. This weightlessness lets you exercise without stressing your joints, making it ideal for people with arthritis. And water resists your movements more than air does, so you can get quite a workout.

Depending on the type of arthritis you have and its severity, you may be able to run in the water, swim, do water exercises, or do water aerobics.

Try running in place in chest-deep water. For more of a challenge, run laps from one side of the shallow end to the other. If the running causes pain, try strapping on a personal flotation device. It may add enough buoyancy to ease the pain.

If you like to swim or want to learn how to swim, work with a swimming instructor to find out which strokes are most comfortable for you. The breaststroke, sidestroke, and elementary backstroke are often good ones for people with arthritis.

Water exercises and water aerobics are designed to increase flexibility and strength while decreasing stiffness and pain. They are best learned through classes.

To find a class, try calling your local YMCA or local chapter of the Arthritis Foundation. Some health clubs, public pools, community centers, and hospitals also offer water exercise and water aerobics classes.

Ask if you can watch a class to see what it's like. If it looks safe, try it. Feel free to modify or omit exercises that are too fast, painful, or risky for you.

If you cannot find a class, go to your local video store. It may have water exercise or water aerobics videos that you can study at home before trying them in a pool.

If you have a pool at home or prefer to work out alone, you can design your own pool exercise program. Try to consult with a physical therapist who can show you the best exercises for your particular type of arthritis. Be sure to keep your pool water temperature in the low 80s. Warmer water may make you overheat, while colder water may draw away too much of your body heat or make your joints ache.

Be careful not to overdo it. It's easy to exercise too hard in the water, because its coolness carries away your body heat. So although you're less likely to overheat, it's harder to tell when you are overdoing it.

Check with your doctor before starting any exercise program. Some exercises may not be safe for your eyes, feet, kidneys, heart, or blood pressure.

• •

I travel a lot. How can I possibly keep up an exercise program?

Traveling can make it hard, but not impossible, to stick to an exercise program. Whether it's a business trip, a long-awaited vacation, or a trip to visit relatives or friends, there are ways to keep in shape when you travel. The key is to do some planning before you even leave home.

EXERCISE 31

Pack a pair of walking shoes and some athletic socks. Walking is easier to squeeze into a busy schedule than most exercises. Also, it can be done in either the city or the country.

Other equipment that you can fit into a tightly packed suitcase includes a swimsuit, a jump rope, or an exercise video. If you are driving to your destination, you can take more exercise equipment with you. For example, you can take racquets and balls, your golf clubs, or your bicycle.

Check out the athletic centers at hotels before booking your room. Some hotels offer a small exercise room (perhaps with a stationary bicycle or weight machine). Some have a swimming pool. Other hotels may offer the use of a nearby health club. If you belong to a national health-club chain, see if you can use the club in the city where you're going.

If you are on a business trip that includes long days of tiring meetings, try getting up a bit earlier so you have time for a walk after breakfast. If you are at a conference, try wearing dressy walking shoes instead of your business shoes. You will be more likely to walk around the exhibit hall and to walk to an outside restaurant instead of eating in the convention center.

If you are taking a vacation, consider taking an active one. Many people have wonderful vacations skiing, hiking, or swimming. If you prefer tamer vacations, touring museums or taking a packaged tour to historic sites will keep you walking every day. Even a luxury vacation can offer some chance for exercise. Many resorts and cruise lines have exercise classes or fitness facilities.

If you are visiting friends or relatives, think about their daily habits and map out a plan. Do they hit the sack soon after supper? Do they lie in bed long after you're up? Will they still be going to work or classes while you're there? These are perfect times to exercise without disrupting your hosts' plans. If you won't have time alone, ask your hosts to leave some space in the schedule so that you can exercise. Or suggest that all of you play some tennis or go to the mall or visit a park.

Chapter three: COPING

So what's wrong with stress, anyway? Everyone I work with is whining about it all the time! I say stress is good! It gets me charged up—for diabetes, or whatever!

You're right, a little stress can be good when it comes to dealing with a short-term crisis. But what your co-workers are whining about is probably long-term stress. Being under unrelenting stress is bad for you, especially if you have diabetes. People with diabetes are harmed by stress and stress hormones in two ways.

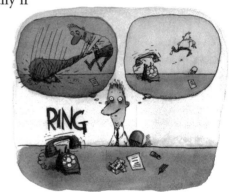

First, being constantly under stress can wear down your immune system or weaken your organs. It can also change the way you respond to future stress. You may get sick more often or even have a heart attack. So you see, stress isn't always good.

Stress can also complicate your diabetes. When you feel stressed, your body gets ready for action. It pumps stress hormones into your blood. Stress hormones make your body release stored glucose and stored fat for extra energy. This extra energy helps your body face up to or run away from the stress. But the extra glucose and fat can only be used by your body if there is enough insulin.

In people with diabetes, there may not be enough insulin. And stress hormones may make it harder for your body to use the insulin that is there. When there is not enough insulin, glucose and fat build up in the blood. High blood glucose and blood fat levels are not good for you.

Second, if you are under stress all the time, you may neglect your diabetes care in order to address the crisis of the day (or week or month). After all, managing your diabetes takes time and effort. If you are constantly putting out fires at work or home, you won't have time to exercise, prepare healthy meals, test your blood glucose, or even see your health care providers on a regular basis.

Try to limit stress to those occasional situations where there is no avoiding it. The rest of the time, find ways to organize your work and personal life so that every day is not frantic.

I'm stressed out all the time, and it hurts my diabetes control. Could biofeedback help?

It is hard to believe that hooking yourself up to a machine that flashes lights and sounds at you can be helpful, but biofeedback can train you to reduce the tension in your muscles. This may help reduce your stress, which may help your diabetes control. Biofeedback will not be a quick fix. But it might pay off big in helping you feel better.

Usually, in biofeedback training, the therapist hooks you up to a machine. The machine measures blood flow, muscle tightness, heart rate, or whatever else you are working on. The machine then provides feedback in the form of lights, sounds, or numbers. For example, the machine might sound a tone when you raise your hand temperature a small amount.

Before you commit to biofeedback, keep in mind that it requires a good bit of effort on your part. As in learning to play an instrument, you must commit yourself to learning the technique, and you must make time for the training and practicing.

To find a certified practitioner of biofeedback in your area or state, send a stamped, self-addressed envelope to the Biofeedback Certification Institute of America, 10200 West 44th Avenue, Suite 304, Wheat Ridge, CO 80033.

I'm 50 years old and I've never kept a New Year's resolution (or any resolution, for that matter). What am I doing wrong?

 Maybe you should try to write down your resolutions *before* opening that New Year's Eve bottle of champagne. Seriously, though, the best way to keep resolutions is to make ones that are easy to keep (no, that is not cheating).

First, write down all your goals for the coming year. Next, take a good, hard look at your list. For each item, ask yourself:

1. Who is this goal for? Did your partner or doctor suggest this goal or is it something you want? It will be a lot easier to stick to a goal *you* want instead of one that is imposed on you by someone else.

2. Is this goal high enough, but not too high? Make goals that push you to perform at a higher level, but that are not unrealistically high.

3. Is this goal practical? Don't sabotage your goal by centering it around something impractical. For example, joining a health club that is inconvenient to reach or selecting equipment that is out of your budget will stall your exercise program before it gets started. You're more likely to follow through if you choose a doable goal.

4. Can you work toward this goal with others? Misery loves company. Find a buddy who can commiserate with you and help keep you going.

The above four questions should weed out goals that would be hard to stick to. Look at the goals that are left. If there are several, choose just one or two. If these turn out to be easy, you can always add more later in the year. But at least you start with a doable goal. Once you've written down your goals, it's time to work on keeping them.

Rewards. Set up a system of rewards for each step toward your goal that you complete. Remind yourself that no one is perfect every hour of every day. Some days, things are going to come up to keep you from working toward your goal. Don't fret over these detours. Just get back on track when you can, and keep your eyes focused forward on your goal, not backward on missteps.

My diabetes is starting to hurt my marriage. I feel that I'm married to my disease rather than my wife. How do I get things back on track?

Diabetes does not make a good marriage partner, so you are wise to want to patch things up with your wife. Here are a few ideas for working through the hard times:

- Tell your partner everything about your diabetes—the good and the bad. Withholding information in an attempt to "protect" your partner will only result in more and more misunderstanding. On the other hand, be careful not to inundate your partner with information. Conveying only your fears and troubles about diabetes will wear out your partner's empathy. Be sure to explain what your limitations are so that your partner will know when you need assistance.

- Help your partner come to grips with your diabetes. Working through the changes brought on by the need to cope with a diabetic partner can be hard. At first, your partner may see you or your diabetes as the bad person and blame you for any disruptions to the relationship. Diabetes-generated problems may make your partner angry or cause your partner to pull away emotionally. Facing problems head on and communicating clearly are keys to helping your partner accept your diabetes.

- Get outside help if you need it. Talk to your friends with diabetes to find out how they solved the problems you are facing. Perhaps they can recommend a therapist.

- Be open to change. Your diabetes may require you to adopt new roles. These changes will make you rethink what's important in your relationship and life and can make you happier and stronger.

- Focus on what's important. Keep the central focus of your relationship on your mutual goals for the future. Plan fun activities on a regular basis. Express your appreciation and love for your partner every day.

Things aren't fun anymore. I don't know whether that's because diabetes is such a drag—or something else. What can you tell me about depression?

Depression does not always feel like sadness. Sometimes it feels like boredom or "nerves" or like there is a 50-pound sack constantly weighing you down. The fact that you feel things aren't fun anymore may mean that you are depressed. Answer the following questions to help you determine whether you are indeed depressed:

- Are things that used to be fun no longer fun?
- Do you have trouble falling asleep, wake up often in the night, or want to sleep a lot more than usual?
- Do you wake up earlier than usual and have trouble falling back to sleep?
- Do you eat more or less than you used to, making you gain or lose weight?
- Do you have trouble paying attention or get distracted easily?
- Do you feel drained of energy?
- Do you often feel nervous or "antsy"?
- Are you less interested in sex?
- Do you cry more often?
- Do you feel you never do anything right or think that you are a burden to other people?
- Do you feel sad or worse in the morning than you do the rest of the day?

- Do you think you would be better off dead? Do you think about hurting yourself or committing suicide?

   If you answered yes to three or more of these questions, or if you answered yes to one or two questions and you have felt this way for 2 weeks or more, you may be depressed. Get help. If you answered yes to the last question, get help right away.

   Depression can be caused by a physical illness, like diabetes. Check with your doctor to see if there is a physical cause for your depression. You may want to see a mental health professional (psychiatrist, psychologist, social worker, or counselor). Treatment may involve counseling or antidepressant medication or both.

- -

 My life is a mess. Half the time, I can't do my blood tests because I can't even find my meter and supplies in all the clutter of my house. How can I get organized for diabetes—and for life?

 Humankind has long known the value of being organized. In the 8th century B.C., Hesiod wrote, "It is best to do things systematically, since we are only human, and disorder is our worst enemy." More than 2,000 years later we are still struggling against clutter and chaos.

   Believe it or not, organization can be easier than you (or Hesiod) think. Here are some simple rules that will help you convert clutter to order and make your life smoother at home and at work:

- Have a place for everything. It's hard to put things away if there's no place they belong. For example, if you're always losing your diabetes pamphlets and books, why not get a file box to put them in?

- Aim for being able to find things, not for being neat. It's better to keep your bills in plain sight than to have a clean desk and overdue payments.

- Don't keep your plan secret. Tell your family about your efforts to be more organized. Put labels on boxes, shelves, file cabinets, and other places so it's always clear to you and others what goes where.

- Store things near where you use them. How often will you test your glucose if you keep your meter on a high shelf in the closet?

- Break chores into parts. Don't set a goal like straightening your whole office or house in 1 day. Instead, choose one drawer or closet to start. Choose another for another day.

- Give yourself a time limit. If you give yourself 1 hour to pick up clutter or organize a closet, you'll be more likely to do it than if you plan not to stop until you drop.

- Rank your chores. Allot the most time—and the time of the day you're at your best—to the most important tasks. Things that are less important don't deserve good time slots.

- Make lists. To-do lists, shopping lists, phone lists, and others can make your life easier.

- Throw away what you don't need. If you can't bear to toss something, think about donating it to a charity or lending it to someone who needs it.

- Decide what to do with mail the first time you look at it. Cut out the middle man (your desk). Sort next to a trash can so you can toss the junk mail immediately.

• •

I'm angry—really, really, angry—about having diabetes. What can I do before I blow up?

Glad you asked. I'd hate for you to do a Mt. St. Helens reenactment. Besides which, if you let anger overwhelm you, it can lead to high blood pressure, high glucose levels, headaches, or depression. Fortunately, you have taken your anger as a sign that something is wrong and seem ready to correct it. Here are 10 tips for dealing with your anger:

COPING 39

1. Defuse it. When you get really ticked off, try talking slowly, taking deep breaths, drinking a glass of water, sitting down, leaning back, and keeping your hands down at your sides.

2. Let it out. Like Mt. St. Helens, sometimes you have to blow. When that happens, do a physical activity like jogging or raking leaves, watch an intense movie, or cry. Write down on a piece of paper what you feel like saying or shouting. Go off by yourself to express your anger, then return to the situation.

3. Ask yourself, how important is it? Will that spilled glass of milk or that traffic jam matter next week? Some things are just too trivial to be worth your anger.

4. Laugh at it. Find something funny about the situation. Sometimes, laughter can push out anger.

5. Let it give you strength. Anger can give you the courage to speak up for yourself or protect someone else.

6. Let it help you grow. Dealing with problems is what makes you wiser, stronger, or better.

7. Learn more about it. Start an anger diary. Write down when you felt angry, where you were, who you were with, why you felt angry, and what you did. After a few weeks, read it over. Try to understand what is making you angry. The better you understand your anger, the better you will be able to deal with it.

8. Accept it as a part of grieving. Many people believe there are five steps to grieving: denial, anger, bargaining, depression, and acceptance. It is normal to get angry as part of grieving about having diabetes. It is also normal to finish being angry and move on with your life.

9. Find the emotion behind your anger. Anger is often the result of another emotion that, for some reason, you find hard to express. Anger can be a response to your grief over having diabetes, but anger may also stem from fear, embarrassment, or pain. Identifying the emotion behind your anger may help you nip your anger in the bud.

10. Get outside help. Counseling can help you find the cause of your anger and learn better responses to it.

On one hand, I feel I should tell people about my diabetes in case I have an emergency. On the other, I feel that my health isn't anyone's business but mine. Do you have advice on whether to tell or not?

Like most things in life, whether to tell or not tell depends on the circumstances. Here are several situations in which you would want to tell—and a few situations in which you might prefer not to:

Reasons To Tell

- You are right to be concerned about an emergency. If you take insulin or sulfonylureas (a class of diabetes pills), you may sometimes have low blood glucose reactions. These can make you so confused that you are unable to help yourself. If people know you have diabetes, they can help you when you have a reaction.

- Being open helps other people learn about diabetes, its symptoms, and treatments. As a result, someone you know may seek early treatment.

- Some people have a hard time accepting they have diabetes. Telling others may help you pass through this stage more easily.

- If you tell everyone, you no longer have to hide a big part of your life. And you don't need to keep track of which people are in the know.

- Telling helps you separate your true friends from the rest.

Clearly, in many situations, it makes a lot of sense to tell. It's safer and often easier. But there may be times when it is just as well not to tell.

COPING 41

Reasons Not To Tell

- In many situations, your diabetes is nobody else's business. Strangers or slight acquaintances don't need to know about it.
- If you don't tell, then you are unlikely ever to lose a promotion or a job because of your diabetes. You have the legal right to wait until after you've been hired to tell about your diabetes. If you use insulin, though, you are legally disqualified from certain jobs (e.g., military service, commercial truck drivers, and commercial pilots). In those cases, of course, you wouldn't want to lie or misrepresent yourself.

Chapter four:
HEALTHY COOKING AND EATING

Everywhere you turn, people are talking about antioxidants. What are they, and do I need to take them?

While they may sound like a gasoline additive ("new ProCare antioxidants protect your engine from corrosion"), antioxidants are actually compounds in foods that may protect your body from oxidation, or so the theory goes.

Oxidation occurs when your body's molecules are attacked by free radicals. While they may sound like revolutionaries recently let out of prison, free radicals are actually by-products of chemical reactions in your body.

Free radicals can damage other molecules and may lead to diseases, such as heart disease and cancer. Antioxidants may protect your molecules from attack by free radicals, thereby helping you fight diseases and even slow aging.

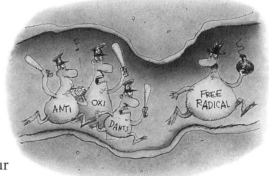

Antioxidants include vitamin C, vitamin E, beta-carotene, and flavonoids. You are probably already getting antioxidants from the foods you eat. But are you getting enough?

HEALTHY COOKING AND EATING 43

The amounts of antioxidants you need for protection from free-radical damage may be higher than the Recommended Dietary Allowances (RDAs). But researchers don't yet know exactly how much you need—or how much is too much.

The best way to increase your intake of antioxidants is to eat more fruits and vegetables. Vitamin C is found in citrus fruits, strawberries, kiwifruit, bell peppers, and broccoli. Carrots, sweet potatoes, spinach, and greens have beta carotene. You can get some vitamin E from apples, mangoes, and blackberries, but you can get more from a tablespoon of vegetable oil or from a couple handfuls of nuts and seeds. One low-fat source of vitamin E is some fortified breakfast cereals.

If you are hoping to take the easy way out by popping vitamin pills, you may be selling yourself short: 1) other nutrients in food may boost the action of antioxidants, and 2) it is likely that other antioxidants have not even been discovered yet.

• •

I'm not a fan of meat, and I'd like to experiment with a vegetarian diet. What should I know?

You should know that there are five kinds of vegetarians: vegan, lacto-vegetarian, ovo-vegetarian, lacto-ovo vegetarian, and semi-vegetarian. The table on p. 45 shows what each kind of vegetarian eats.

You should also know that a vegetarian diet may have a positive effect on your diabetes. If you have type 1 diabetes, you may find you need less insulin. If you have type 2 diabetes, you may start to lose weight, which can improve your blood glucose control.

Before you cross over to a vegetarian diet, discuss your decision with your dietitian. Your dietitian can help you substitute foods for those you want to take out of your meal plan and make sure you get the nutrients that your body needs.

Not surprisingly, leaving meat out of your diet leaves some nutritional holes that you need to fill in other ways. The American Dietetic Association advises vegetarians to

Types of Vegetarians

	Eats	Does Not Eat
Vegan	Fruits, vegetables, legumes, grains, nuts, seeds	Meat, fish, shellfish, poultry, dairy products, eggs
Lacto-Vegetarian	Fruits, vegetables, legumes, grains, nuts, seeds, dairy products	Meat, fish, shellfish, poultry, eggs
Ovo-Vegetarian	Fruits, vegetables, legumes, grains, nuts, seeds, eggs	Meat, fish, shellfish, poultry, dairy products
Lacto-Ovo Vegetarian	Fruits, vegetables, legumes, grains, nuts, seeds, eggs, dairy products	Meat, fish, shellfish, poultry
Semi-Vegetarian	Fruits, vegetables, legumes, grains, nuts, seeds, eggs, dairy products, fish, shellfish, poultry	Meat

- Eat foods rich in vitamin C for better absorption of the iron in foods.
- Eat whole-grain rather than refined foods.
- Get protein from grains, legumes, or low-fat dairy products.
- Eat no more than 3 or 4 egg yolks a week.
- Have a source of vitamin B_{12} if you eat no animal products at all. For example, eat a cereal with added B_{12} or take a vitamin B_{12} pill.

Some people say that sugar is like poison for people with diabetes. Others say it's no big deal. Who's right?

They're both wrong. Sugar is neither poison nor of so little consequence that it can be regarded as "no big deal." Sugar is one of the two major types of carbohydrate. The other major type is starch. Sugars and starches raise your blood glucose level. People who say that sugar is like poison for people with diabetes probably think that sugars raise your blood glucose level faster than starches or other carbohydrates. But this is not the case. Research has shown that sugars do not raise your blood glucose level any more than starches or other carbohydrates.

These people may also think that fructose, a sugar found in fruits and vegetables, is better for them than other sugars. Although fructose may cause a smaller rise in your blood glucose level than other sugars, large amounts of fructose may increase your cholesterol levels. So there is no reason to use fructose in place of other sugars. There is also no advantage to using fruit juice or fruit juice concentrates in place of other sugars. They provide the same amount of calories, and they raise blood glucose about as high as other sugars do.

The people who say that sugar is no big deal may think that they can just go ahead and start shoveling sugar over their Cocoa Puffs. But—and this is a big but—you can't simply add foods with sugar to your meals. You must substitute foods with sugar for other carbohydrates in your meal plan. Your dietitian can help you figure out how to do this. Just keep in mind that sugars average about 16 calories per teaspoon. And often, foods high in sugar are also high in fat—a double whammy.

Sugar substitutes, on the other hand, are free foods; you can add them to your meal plan without taking anything else out. The American Diabetes Association still says aspartame (Nutrasweet, Equal), saccharin (Sweet'n Low, Sugar Twin, or Sweet 10), and acesulfame potassium (Sweet One or Sunette) are safe in moderate amounts.

I keep hearing about "Exchanges." What are they, and what do they have to do with me?

Diabetes exchanges are lists of foods grouped together because they are alike. One serving of any of the foods on a list has about the same amount of carbohydrate, protein, fat, and calories. Any food on a list may be "exchanged" or traded for any other food on the same list.

Exchange lists are used for making meal plans for people with diabetes. Using exchange lists, your dietitian will help you make a master menu. It will tell you the number of food exchanges to eat at each meal and snack. You then choose foods that add up to those exchanges.

With the exchange lists, you don't need to count calories or fat grams. You don't need to guess the percentages of various nutrients. As long as you follow your master menu, you are eating a balanced diet. In other words, you can take that calculator out of your kitchen (but you may still need the scale to measure portion sizes).

In *Exchange Lists for Meal Planning*, published by the American Diabetes Association and The American Dietetic Association, there are 15 exchange lists:

Carbohydrates

1. Starch List
2. Fruit List
3. Milk List
4. Other Carbohydrates List
5. Vegetable List

Meat and Meat Substitutes

6. Very-Lean List
7. Lean List
8. Medium-Fat List
9. High-Fat List

Fats

10. Monounsaturated Fats List
11. Polyunsaturated Fats List
12. Saturated Fats List

Other Lists

13. Free Foods List
14. Combination Foods List
15. Fast Foods List

HEALTHY COOKING AND EATING 47

I love salt in my food. I mean, L-O-V-E it! Unfortunately, my doctor says I should cut back even though I don't have high blood pressure. Can't I sneak in a few shakes now and then?

You can sneak a few shakes of salt now and then as long as you get no more than about 2,400 milligrams of sodium a day. That's a little more than a teaspoon of salt. Most doctors believe people with normal blood pressure should observe this limit. Since you are such a big salt lover, you are probably over the 2,400 milligram a day limit. Most Americans are. People need only about 500 milligrams of sodium each day, but the average American eats 8 times that much.

Most of the salt in our diets comes from the salt added to processed and prepared foods. Foods high in salt include canned foods, cured and smoked meats (bacon, sausage, salami, hot dogs, bologna), pickles, salad dressings, mustard, ketchup, soy sauce, breakfast cereals, cheese, frozen dinners, and salty snacks.

When buying these and other prepared foods, choose those with the least sodium. Many are marked as low-sodium, reduced-sodium, or unsalted. Here are some other ways to reduce your sodium intake:

- Skip the salt when cooking. (Note, however, that some baking recipes, such as those made with yeast, need salt for the recipe to work.)
- Jazz up your food with other flavors. Try lemon juice, flavored vinegars, peppers, garlic, onions, salt-free seasoning blends, and other herbs and spices in place of salt.
- Rinse salted canned foods (vegetables, beans, fish, shellfish, and meats) with cold water for 1 minute to remove some of the sodium.
- Substitute chicken or turkey for prosciutto, ham, or other salty cured meats.

Since you're used to eating very salty foods, your less salty foods may taste odd when you first cut back. But after a few weeks, you'll start noticing and enjoying all the flavors that had been buried by the salt.

Would you please give me some easy ways to cut fat from my diet?

Cutting fat from your diet can be easier than you think. There are many small things you can do that add up to big improvements. Here are 20:

1. Buy lean cuts of meat, such as top round steak, eye round roast, pork tenderloin, lamb shank, and veal leg. Try game meats, like venison and rabbit. These tend to be leaner than other meats.

2. Avoid cured or smoked meats, including hot dogs, salami, bologna, bacon, and sausage. These tend to be higher in fat.

3. Choose unbreaded plain fresh or frozen fish and canned fish packed in water. Or, rinse oil-packed fish under running water to remove the added vegetable oil.

4. Look for ground chicken or turkey with less than 7 to 8% fat by weight (36% or less of its calories from fat).

5. Trim fat from meat and take skin off poultry either before or after cooking.

6. Marinate meats and vegetables in lemon juice, lime juice, sherry, wine, vinegar, low-fat or nonfat broth, or vegetable juice instead of oil.

7. Use nonstick cookware, so you won't need to use as much fat.

8. Cook food in a tablespoon or less of an unsaturated oil, such as olive or canola.

9. Use unsaturated oils in place of butter or margarine.

10. Choose soft tub, liquid, light, or diet margarine that is labeled low in *trans* fatty acids.

HEALTHY COOKING AND EATING 49

11. Baste with broth, vegetable or fruit juice, or wine rather than with pan drippings.

12. Microwave onions, garlic, peppers, and other vegetables in a bit of water instead of sautéing them in oil.

13. Skim the fat from soups, stews, broths, gravies, and sauces. Chilling the food in the refrigerator until the fat floats on top and hardens makes the fat easier to remove.

14. Top baked potatoes, air-popped popcorn, or roast turkey or chicken with butter-flavored nonstick vegetable oil spray instead of butter or margarine.

15. Switch to low-fat or nonfat versions of your favorite foods.

16. Use skim milk, 1% milk, or buttermilk made from skim milk instead of whole or 2% milk.

17. Choose low-fat or nonfat yogurt, sour cream, mayonnaise, salad dressings, and cheeses.

18. When you make a pie, use only a single crust. When possible, make a crumb crust instead of a pastry crust.

19. Use two egg whites in place of one whole egg in egg dishes and other recipes.

20. In muffin recipes, try substituting nonfat yogurt for the oil and eggs.

• •

My supermarket has starting carrying supplements called "phytochemicals." Because these come from vegetables, they must be safe and good for you. Should I take them—especially considering that I hate vegetables?

Sorry, you are going to have to keep forcing down those vegetables. Phytochemicals may sound great, but there are many reasons not to take them—at least not yet.

- First, it's much more fun to get your phytochemicals by eating tasty foods than by taking a pill. Although you don't like vegetables, you can still get phytochemicals from fruits, nuts, whole grains, and herbs and spices. Eating many different

50 Dear Diabetes Advisor

kinds of foods will help you take in a wide variety of phytochemicals.

- Second, pills can be costly. It's usually cheaper to get your phytochemicals from your everyday diet.

- Third, certain phytochemicals may work best when combined with other nutrients. You might only receive their full benefit when you eat them in a food.

- Fourth, research on phytochemicals is still in the early stages. No one yet knows what all the phytochemicals are, let alone how they work or how much you need of each. If you take a pill, you may miss out on some good phytochemicals, and you may take in too-high levels of others.

If for some reason you still decide to take phytochemicals, check with your doctor first.

Coffee's a free food, right? So does that mean I can order a mocha latte grande and not worry?

Sorry, your flavored latte (coffee with milk) may not be okay. Flavored coffees may sound exotic, but they're really just another form of American junk food.

Sugar is the main ingredient of flavored coffees. Corn syrup (another form of sugar) is usually also near the top of the list. The fat content can be very high—from 1 to 3.5 grams per serving, depending on the flavor and brand.

You'll need to count that extra fat and sugar (unless you opt for a nonfat, sugar-free version) in your meal plan.

Coffee is only a free food when you drink it black, or with a sugar substitute, and/or with a nondairy creamer (liquid, 1 Tbsp; powdered, 2 tsp).

If you're a coffee lover, there are more healthful ways to be adventuresome. Gourmet coffee stores sell beans from many

HEALTHY COOKING AND EATING 51

countries. You can also try foreign brewing methods, such as espresso, that make coffee taste exotic.

I keep hearing chromium supplements can help people with type 2 diabetes. True?

It's true for certain people and false for others. Chromium supplements can help people with type 2 diabetes who have a chromium deficiency. A chromium deficiency can cause higher blood glucose and blood fat levels and impaired glucose tolerance.

If a lab test (it's quite expensive) shows that you have a chromium deficiency, your doctor may have you take a chromium supplement. If you already get enough chromium, taking extra will not help your blood glucose or blood fat levels.

Most people with diabetes do get enough chromium. The recommended safe and adequate intake of chromium is just 50 to 200 micrograms a day. One microgram is one-millionth of a gram, and one gram is equal to one-twenty-eighth of an ounce. So, this is a small amount.

If you are concerned about getting enough chromium or want to boost your intake, try eating foods high in chromium, such as wheat germ, Brewer's yeast, whole grains, and liver. Seafood and potatoes are also good sources of chromium.

I have no time to cook healthy meals. Aren't there convenience foods that are good for you?

Absolutely. Here's how to pick out the good convenience foods. First, look at the food label. Do you want to put these ingredients in your body? Sometimes, manufacturers can only give food a long shelf life by adding lots of sugar, salt, or preservatives. Are the Nutrition Facts in line with your healthy eating plan?

Next, look at the price. Most convenience foods cost more than making the food from scratch. Is the time you will save worth the extra cost? If the food passes these two tests, then it's ready for a road test. Take it home and try it out. Check the label for hints on making the best of the new food. Now check out these 10 good convenience foods that deserve to be staples in your kitchen:

1. **Bread.** Store-bought bread is usually cheaper and less time-consuming than making it yourself.
2. **Chopped frozen onions.** Great for stews, casseroles, and other dishes with long cooking times. Not as good for sautéing, but try simmering them in a bit of wine or broth first.
3. **Minced garlic in jars.** Use as you would fresh garlic.
4. **Frozen vegetables.** Use when you can't find fresh, ripe veggies. Choose those without sauces.
5. **Canned tomatoes.** Often of higher quality than fresh tomatoes picked green and shipped long distance to get to you. Plus, you avoid the time it takes to peel fresh tomatoes.
6. **Bags of baby or baby-cut carrots.** They make a perfect snack or cheerful addition to a relish tray.
7. **Skinless chicken pieces.** How often have you left the fatty skin on chicken rather than take the time to wrestle it off? Skinless chicken pieces are ready to go into your recipe with no chopping or pulling.
8. **Canned beans.** Even though dry beans are easy to cook, you do have to plan ahead. Canned beans let you delay your dinner decision till the last minute.
9. **Grated parmesan cheese.** Easier than grating it yourself.
10. **Nonstick cooking spray.** Look for sprays that are entirely canola or olive oil. Aerosols coat less heavily (and so add fewer calories) than pump sprays.

I have diabetes, so should I eat "dietetic" foods?

Although "diabetic" and "dietetic" sound similar, they are not closely related. They are more like second cousins. Whether dietetic foods are worthwhile for someone with diabetes depends on why you are eating them and whether they are providing what you thought you were getting.

- **Reduced-calorie.** To lose weight, people must take in fewer calories than they use. So it makes sense that reduced-calorie foods would help with weight loss. But some people who eat reduced-calorie foods end up eating extra calories at other times to make up for the reduced-calorie food. Look hard at your own eating habits. Are you truly taking in fewer calories on days you eat reduced-calorie foods? Or do you get hungry faster and then eat more to fill back up?

- **Sugar-free.** Although you do not need to avoid sugar, you may want to eat sugar-free foods as a way of cutting calories. If so, keep in mind that some "sugar-free" foods contain honey, fructose, or molasses. These foods may have just as many calories as the regular versions.

- **Low-fat or nonfat.** If you're looking to lose weight, watch out. Some low-fat foods have just as many calories as full-fat foods! Their makers add extra sugar to make up for the loss of fat flavor. Also, some foods, like cheeses, have so much fat that reduced-fat versions are still pretty fatty. To make sure you know what you are getting, read the Nutrition Facts label.

- **Low-salt or no-salt.** For some people, eating too much salt can raise their blood pressure. If salt does not raise your blood pressure and your doctor has not told you to avoid sodium, compare the low-salt and full-salt versions of a food, and buy the one that tastes the best to you.

Before buying a dietetic food, compare its ingredients, nutrients, and price with other brands of similar foods. Make sure the food really does give you what you want. If you are trying to lose weight, pick a food that is low in calories. If you are trying to keep your heart healthy, pick a food that is low in both overall fat and saturated fat. Don't be fooled by foods that imply they are healthier but whose nutrient list tells a different story.

I eat fast food a lot, but I always feel guilty because my doctor says it's bad for me. How can I get a good fast-food meal?

While it's possible to eat an entire day's worth of fat, salt, and calories in just one fast-food meal, today's fast-food restaurants are offering healthier choices. Fast-food places that are proud of their new healthier choices often have nutrition sheets. Look for foods high in nutrients and low in fat. With a little care, you can fit a fast-food meal into your healthy eating plan. Here's how to order sensibly:

- For breakfast, try a plain bagel, toast, or English muffin. Drink low-fat (1%) milk. Order cold cereal with skim milk, oatmeal, or plain scrambled eggs. Avoid bacon and sausage.
- Load up on lettuce and vegetables at the salad bar. Go easy on the bacon bits, cheeses, olives, croutons, mayonnaise, macaroni salads, and dressing (too much of even a low-calorie salad dressing can make a difference).
- Order regular or junior-size sandwiches rather than the larger "jumbo," "giant," or "deluxe" sandwiches to get fewer calories and less fat, cholesterol, and sodium.
- Choose plain lean roast beef, turkey or chicken breast, or lean ham sandwiches.
- Skip the croissant and eat your sandwich on a bun or bread instead to save calories and fat.

HEALTHY COOKING AND EATING

- Choose plain chicken or fish that is roasted, grilled, baked, or broiled without fat. Chicken or fish that is battered, breaded, or fried is higher in calories and fat.

- Order items plain without cheese, sauces, mayonnaise, or other toppings. Add lettuce, tomato, onion, salsa, or mustard instead.

- Choose cheese pizza with vegetables. Other toppings, such as pepperoni, sausage, olives, and extra cheese, add calories, fat, and sodium.

- Order nonfried items when eating Mexican fast foods. Choose chicken over beef. Avoid beans refried in lard. Pile on extra lettuce, tomatoes, and salsa. Go easy on cheese, sour cream, and guacamole. Watch out for the deep-fried taco salad shell—a taco salad can have more than 1,000 calories!

- If you have room for dessert, go for sugar-free nonfat frozen yogurt. Ices, sorbets, and sherbets have less fat and fewer calories than ice cream, but the sugar they contain needs to be factored into your meal plan. Some places now offer fresh fruit!

• •

 Do I need to take minerals? My doctor says no, but many of my friends with diabetes take them.

 Peer pressure is hard to resist, but your doctor probably knows your needs best. Your friends may be taking mineral supplements because their doctor has found they lack enough of a certain mineral. Or they may fall into one of the categories below:

- **Dieters.** People who take in fewer than 1,200 calories each day may need iron and folate.

- **Vegetarians.** People who eat no animal foods at all may need vitamin B_{12}, calcium, iron, vitamin B_2 (riboflavin), and zinc.

- **People at risk for bone diseases.** People at risk for bone diseases may need vitamin D, calcium, and magnesium.

- **Elderly.** People over 65 may need calcium and folate.
- **Pregnant or breastfeeding women.** Pregnant or breastfeeding women may need extra iron, zinc, calcium, and folate.
- **People who take diuretics.** People who take diuretics (water pills) may need magnesium, calcium, potassium, and zinc.
- **People who have foot ulcers.** People who have foot ulcers may need zinc.

Most people won't be harmed by taking a multivitamin with minerals. Still, it's not a good idea to take large doses of minerals in the hope that one turns out to be useful. Some minerals are harmful in large amounts. Check with your doctor before taking any supplement. And tell your friends to do the same.

I've been looking at bottled waters and finding all sorts of things in them in addition to water—things like sugar and salt. What's the story? When did water stop being just water?

Variety is the spice of life, and apparently that now applies to water as well. As concerns about the safety of tap water have increased, bottled water's popularity has risen accordingly. To keep their customers interested, bottled water providers have developed different flavors and types of water.

- **Mineral water.** Mineral water has minerals like calcium and magnesium dissolved in it.
- **Sparkling water.** Sparkling water contains carbon dioxide bubbles. The bubbles flavor the water and make it sparkly, like a soft drink.
- **Spring water.** Spring water comes from underground springs.
- **Seltzer.** Seltzer is sparkling water made from filtered tap water.
- **Club soda.** Club soda is seltzer with added minerals.

HEALTHY COOKING AND EATING 57

Some people enjoy drinking bottled waters because of the variety. Those different tastes make it easier to take in 6 to 8 cups a day. But before you overindulge, take a look at the ingredient list on the label to find out what else you are getting with your water.

- **Sugar.** It's hard to think of a product that needs sweetening less than water. Yet, some seltzers and club sodas do contain sugar.
- **Salt.** Water with minerals or added carbonation may be high in sodium. If you are watching your salt intake, buy waters with little or no sodium.
- **Minerals.** Some people love the taste of minerals; some hate it. Try several brands to find a mineral content that is to your liking.
- **Source.** The water's label usually tells you where the water comes from. It may be a natural source, such as a spring. Or it may be a city water supply—that is, tap water.

I may go crazy if I can't have some of my favorite foods—like chocolate. Most of the time fresh fruit will do, but sometimes I just need to feed a special craving. How can I do this and still stay healthy?

It may seem that eating a healthful diet means saying no to the foods you like best. But it's okay to give in to your urges sometimes. Here are a few foods many people crave and ways you can indulge these cravings healthfully.

- **Chocolate.** Like the mythical sirens luring sailors toward a rocky shore, chocolate seems to cry out to be eaten. Fortunately, you can get a chocolate infusion without wrecking your health. Look for recipes that call for little added fat and for cocoa powder instead of chocolate. Cocoa powder has far less fat than chocolate. Yet, brownies, cakes, puddings, and hot chocolate made with cocoa have a deep chocolate flavor. Plus, cocoa is easier to cook with than finicky chocolate. Another option is sugar-free chocolate-flavored soft drinks. These low-fat drinks offer another way to get chocolate flavor without added fat and sugar.

- **Ice cream.** True, it's not healthy to indulge in Ben & Jerry's Cherry Garcia every day, but there are several kinds of luscious low-fat and fat-free frozen desserts (fruit sherbets, frozen yogurts, and ice creams) available at your grocery store. But read the label before trying a new dessert. Sometimes, the product will contain lots of extra sugar (and calories) to make up for the lower fat.

- **Snack foods.** Most stores now carry reduced-fat and low-fat chips, crackers, and cookies. There are also unsalted, low-salt, and sugar-free versions.

Work with your dietitian to make room in your meal plan for your cravings.

Chapter five: WEIGHT LOSS

I want to lose weight. Please don't tell me to diet and exercise. I've tried that—many times. Couldn't I just take one of those pills for losing weight?

Sure, you could take a pill for weight loss. But it may or may not help you lose weight. Some people taking weight-loss pills don't lose any weight at all! Others lose 10 percent or less of their body weight. For example, a 200-pound person might lose 20 pounds. Losing 10 percent can be helpful to you, though. Your glucose level may drop, your blood pressure may drop, your cholesterol level may improve, and your joints may hurt less.

Even if weight-loss pills do work for you, most doctors believe only people who are obese or who have health problems caused by being overweight should take weight-loss drugs.

Weight-loss drugs act by changing the levels of nervous system chemicals, such as catecholamines and serotonin, in your body. These chemicals control your appetite. However, the changes to your body chemistry are not permanent. Once you stop taking the weight-loss drugs, your appetite returns. When appetite returns, pounds are likely to as well.

Because weight-loss pills make you feel less hungry, it's easier to stick to a low-calorie eating plan. But if you eat just as much as before and don't exercise, you won't lose weight.

WEIGHT LOSS 61

All weight-loss drugs have side effects and can affect blood glucose levels. So it's safer to regard weight-loss drugs as short-term helpers rather than as long-term solutions for a weight problem.

The best way to achieve permanent weight loss is through an exercise program, an eating plan for weight loss, and behavior modification (learning new habits).

I'm seeing ads for weight-loss programs that have many clients who have lost weight. I've tried losing weight myself and failed. Now I think a program might help. How do I choose one?

Don't you just love those ads where the now svelte woman holds up the huge pair of pants she used to wear before she started the weight-loss program? Doesn't it just make you want to run out and sign up? As with all advertisements that promise you big returns if you pay up, weight-loss center advertisements try to lure you in with promises of painless, dramatic success. Sorry, but that isn't always the case.

Some programs are based on sound ideas, while others are one step shy of quackery. A good program includes exercise, education about food and nutrition, a balanced diet, and behavior modification (that is, learning new habits). Some even have follow-up programs to help you maintain your weight loss. Beware a program that implies it's 100 percent safe or promises lots of weight loss in a short amount of time. Weight loss should be fairly slow—no more than 1 to 2 pounds a week—to be safe.

Be sure the program has a medical doctor, physician's assistant, or nurse practitioner, and a psychologist and an exercise physiologist on staff. Look for a program that specializes in helping people with diabetes. Once you've found some programs you might join, be sure to ask lots of questions, such as

- How much does your program cost?
- What does that cost cover?
- Are there extra costs for vitamins, cassette tapes, or other items?
- Do I need to buy your program's food?
- How does your diet stack up against the *Dietary Guidelines for Americans*?
- Who staffs your program?
- What are their credentials?
- How would your program help me lose weight?
- How do you adapt your plan for people with diabetes?
- What are the risks of your program?
- What kind of maintenance program do you offer?

• •

My doctor says to lose weight. Easy for him to say! He says I should weigh what I did when I was young. I tell him, "Yeah, right!" How do I set a goal I might reach in my lifetime?

Your doctor said you should weigh what you did when you were young?! What age exactly—10, 15, 20? You are right to want to set a realistic goal. Here are things to consider when trying to determine your personal weight-loss goal:

- Compare your weight to the chart of acceptable weights for men and women on p. 64. Now just because you fall below or above the range for your height doesn't mean you have to gain or lose weight. And just because you fall within the range does not mean you are at your best weight. The table just gives you an idea of what a good weight is for a typical person of your height.

- Figure out your body mass index, or BMI. To figure out your BMI, multiply your weight in pounds by 705. Divide this answer by your height in inches. Now divide by your height

WEIGHT LOSS 63

Height and Weight Table for Men and Women

Height without Shoes (feet and inches)	Weight without Clothes (pounds)
4'10"	91–119
4'11"	94–124
5'0"	97–128
5'1"	101–132
5'2"	104–137
5'3"	107–141
5'4"	111–146
5'5"	114–150
5'6"	118–155
5'7"	121–160
5'8"	125–164
5'9"	129–169
5'10"	132–174
5'11"	136–179
6'0"	140–184
6'1"	144–189
6'2"	148–195
6'3"	152–200
6'4"	156–205
6'5"	160–211
6'6"	164–216

From the United States Department of Agriculture: *Report of the Dietary Guidelines Advisory Committee on the Dietary Guidelines for Americans,* 1995, p. 10.

again. The answer is your BMI. If you are age 34 or younger, a BMI of 25 and above is considered overweight. If you are 35 or older, a BMI of 27 and above is considered overweight.

- Consider your muscle mass. Muscle weighs a lot. If you are very muscular, a high target weight may be okay. But if you are very flabby, a low target weight may be better.

- Consider your frame size. Bone is heavy. The smaller your bones, the lighter a weight to aim for.
- Consider where your fat is located. Fat on the abdomen, waist, and upper body (apple-shaped body) is less healthy than fat on the hips and thighs (pear-shaped body). A person with a spare tire may need to take off pounds, even if he or she is within the suggested weight range.
- Consider any weight-related health problems you may have. If you have arthritis in your knees or you've had a heart or gallbladder attack, being overweight has already been a big burden to you. You may want to set a lower target than someone who has suffered few bad effects from being overweight.

• •

 I'm a middle-aged man who's getting pretty thick around the middle. I'd like to lose weight—and shape up at the same time. Could I use weights to lose weight?

 Because you asked so nicely, I'm going to give you the weight-loss secret: To lose the most weight, do both aerobic exercises and strength exercises.

Aerobic exercises burn calories fast. Plus, as you get fitter, you can exercise harder and burn more calories. Strength exercises shape your muscles so that you look thinner. Plus, the muscles you get will burn more calories than the fat you had.

To lose 1 pound by exercise, you need to burn 3,500 more calories than you take in. The more you weigh, the more calories you burn per minute. Someone who weighs about 200 pounds burns 12 to 20 calories per minute walking briskly.

Different exercises burn different numbers of calories per minute. Contrary to what you might think, the best exercises for losing weight are not those that burn the most calories per minute. The reason: You cannot keep up the pace very long. It's better to pick an easier exercise that you can keep up for 30 to 60 minutes, because the longer you exercise, the more calories you burn.

For the first few months, you won't lose much weight. Don't feel bad. As your lungs and heart get stronger, you will be able to exert more effort and use more calories. Your muscles will also get bigger. Then they will burn more calories—even while you're sleeping! As you build muscle and become sleeker, you will see drops in your measurements before you lose weight.

Check with your doctor before starting any exercise program. Some exercises may not be safe for your eyes, feet, kidneys, heart, or blood pressure.

I keep reading that dieting is out. But I'm still fat. Why shouldn't I diet to lose weight?

You don't really want to diet do you? Think of the hunger, guilt, and ultimate sense of failure when you regain all of the weight you suffered so much to lose. Do you really want that again?

The fact is, cutting back on food temporarily—dieting—rarely works. The only way to lose weight and keep it off is to exercise more, eat less (fewer calories), and adopt healthful eating habits. Healthful eating habits mean eating food that is low in fat, high in starches and fiber, and moderate in protein, sodium, and sugars. Here are some reasons why dieting fails:

- Dieting just doesn't work over the long term. It's hard to keep it up long enough to lose the weight you want. Plus, once you stop, it's natural to go back to the bad eating habits that made you overweight in the first place. Then you'll gain the weight right back.

- Dieting is punishing; good eating habits are rewarding. Dieting forces you to face a future without foods and treats that you love (no more Oreos dunked in chocolate milk). But a thought-out, healthful eating plan makes room for treats.

- Dieting is not always good for you. It can lead to eating disorders and depression, among other ills. But a low-fat eating plan high in vegetables, fruits, grains, and legumes reduces your cholesterol level and protects you against heart disease and many forms of cancer.

- Dieting makes your body think it is starving. Severe calorie cutting slows your body's metabolism (making it hard to lose weight). Your body signals its distress with hunger pangs, so you'll eat more. Is this any way to treat yourself?
- Dieting makes you feel guilty. Either you feel guilty because you don't sample some special treat your friend makes or you feel guilty because you do sample the treat. Healthful eating habits are not about rules and prohibitions.
- Dieting focuses your attention on the wrong goals: getting the fewest calories or losing the most pounds. But good eating habits give you a more healthful goal: getting the most nutrition from the calories you do eat.

I'm trying so hard to lose weight. What foods are best for weight loss?

Now you're talking. Stick to eating healthful foods. To lose weight, you'll do best cutting down on calories from fat. Each gram of fat has more than twice as many calories as a gram of carbohydrate or protein. By shifting your diet from fat to carbohydrate and protein, you should be able to eat the same amount of food but take in far fewer calories. Try these nutrition-rich, low-fat foods:

- **Bread.** Good bread is great plain. Go for breads that list whole grains or multigrains as the first ingredient on the label, with 2 to 3 grams of fiber, 1 gram of fat or less, and 80 calories per slice.
- **Pasta.** Pasta is so versatile. When buying premade pasta, look for those made without eggs or oil for the least fat. When making your own, choose recipes with little added oil—and use olive oil.

WEIGHT LOSS 67

- **Cereals.** Choose cereals listing whole grains as the first ingredient on the label. Look for breakfast cereals that have

    No more than 2 grams of fat per serving
    No more than 6 grams of sugars per serving
    Less than 150 calories per serving
    Less than 400 milligrams of sodium per serving
    At least 4 grams of fiber per serving

- **Grains.** There are so many grains to try: wheat, rice, oats, barley, buckwheat groats, bulgur wheat, bran, wheat germ, couscous, quinoa, and amaranth. Most whole grains contain little fat and 100 calories per 1/2 cup of cooked grain. Try them in soups and casseroles and as bases for toppings.

- **Legumes.** Legumes include beans, peas, and lentils. These high-fiber, low-fat sources of protein make a perfect topping for grains or replacement for meat in soups and casseroles. Buy dried beans and lentils, fresh or frozen peas, and fat-free or low-fat varieties of canned beans.

- **Potatoes.** Your basic spud contains no fat. To keep it that way, go for low-fat toppings like nonfat yogurt, low-fat cottage cheese, fat-free sour cream, or salsa.

- **Vegetables.** Wouldn't you know it. The vegetables many of us love to hate are among the best things we can eat. Buy fresh, frozen (without sauces), or canned vegetables.

- **Fruits.** Thank goodness most fruits are excellent foods for weight loss. Buy fresh, frozen (without added sugar), or canned (in water or juice) fruit.

- **Skim milk and milk products.** Nonfat and low-fat are the keys words for yogurt, cheeses, and other dairy foods.

Chapter six:
INSURANCE

 I swear that you need a PhD and then some to understand an insurance statement. What do all those terms mean?

 Actually, you need an HdIJ (higher degree in insurance jargon). Yes, the insurance community has its own language, and you are wise to want to learn it. Here are some of the most common terms you will come across:

- **Covered charge.** Your health insurance company will pay for some charges and not for others. Those that it does pay for are known as "covered charges" or "eligible expenses." Your insurance policy or plan booklet lists what is covered.

- **Deductible.** You may have to pay a certain amount of money each year before your insurance kicks in. For example, your individual deductible may be $250. After you've submitted $250 worth of covered charges, the insurance company will start paying for covered charges. Your family deductible is the charges your whole family has to submit before the insurance company pays bills for family members who have not met their individual deductibles.

- **Co-payment.** In some insurance plans, you must pay a percentage of each bill, even if you have met your deductible.

- **Dependent.** A dependent is a person whom you elect to have covered by your health insurance plan. It may include your husband or wife and your children.
- **EOB.** EOB stands for Explanation of Benefits. This is the form your insurance company sends you listing what charges were submitted to it and what action it is taking on each. Reading these is an art form in itself.
- **Stoploss.** Stoploss is a cutoff point after which all your charges are covered. Once your covered charges for 1 year reach a predetermined figure, such as $10,000, the insurance company will pay all other covered charges for the rest of the year, even if you would normally owe a co-payment. This protects you from catastrophic losses.

If you encounter another term that baffles you, don't be shy about asking for an explanation. It's better to be safe than sorry when it comes to your health insurance coverage.

• •

I've been looking into joining a managed care plan, but some people I know have had bad luck with them. What should I look—and look out—for in a managed care plan?

Managed care plans promise to take care of your health with fewer hassles and costs than traditional health plans. Some keep these promises—and some don't.

Managed care plans try to keep costs under control. Good plans do so by helping you stay healthy and taking care of small problems before they turn into large ones. Bad plans save money by being stingy with care.

Because you have diabetes, it pays to be extra careful when choosing health plans. Here are some questions you'll want to ask to head off unhappy surprises later:

- Does the plan cover diabetes education? The more you know about diabetes, the better you can take care of yourself and the healthier you'll be. So over the long term, diabetes education saves money.

- Does the plan cover basic diabetes supplies? Find out whether the medications (insulin, diabetes pills) and medical supplies (syringes, pumps, test strips) you use to keep your blood glucose in line are covered.

- Does the plan allow your diabetes doctor to send you to the specialists you need? See if you can choose your diabetes doctor as your primary care provider. If not, you may be stuck returning again and again to your primary care provider to ask for referrals. Worse yet, some plans require primary care providers to receive approval from the plan before referring you.

- Does the plan restrict the number of times you can see your diabetes doctor or a specialist during the year? In a year, you may need to see your diabetes doctor, an eye doctor, a foot doctor, a dietitian, and other specialists. Make sure that you are allowed enough visits that you won't run out of care midway through the year.

- Does the plan pay providers a flat fee or a fee for each service they provide? If your provider gets a fee for each service, you might receive unnecessary tests and procedures. On the other hand, if your provider receives a flat fee per patient per year, be aware that such a payment plan gives your provider a financial reason to scrimp on your care.

• •

I really should see a dietitian for advice on my meal plan, but they cost so much. How can I get insurance to pay for a visit?

Ah, insurance companies. You can't live with them, you can't live without them. You may be lucky enough to have an insurance policy that will cover a visit to a dietitian without fussing.

INSURANCE 71

If, however, your insurance company balks at paying, taking the following steps may convince them to cover the cost:

- Contact your state insurance department. Each state has its own laws and regulations governing insurance. More and more states have laws that make insurance companies pay for dietary visits.

- Call your insurance company. Find out what your policy covers. If they do cover visits with a dietitian, be sure to ask what paperwork you need to provide to them.

- Submit a claim each time. Whether your insurance company tells you it will pay or not, submit a claim after each visit to the dietitian. Include 1) a written prescription from your doctor that uses fancy-sounding language like "medical and nutrition therapy for diabetes management" rather than just "nutrition counseling" or "nutrition education" and 2) a letter from your registered dietitian (RD) telling why your visit was medically necessary.

- If turned down again, ask for your claim to be reviewed. Many insurance companies have a review process for disputed claims.

- Consider changing insurance policies or companies, if possible. If your insurance policy won't pay for you to visit a dietitian, it may not pay for other important care you need either.

• •

I signed up for a new health insurance plan that sounded great. Then, when I tried to go for counseling to help me cope with my diabetes, I found out that this plan pays almost nothing for mental health benefits. Next time, what should I look for in a plan?

The next time you look for an insurance plan, find the answers to these questions:

- What problems are considered mental health problems? Insurance plans may classify some brain illnesses, such as manic depression and schizophrenia, as mental problems and other brain illnesses, such as epilepsy, as medical problems.

- What mental health problems are covered? Look at the schedule of benefits to see if mental health problems are covered. Also check the lists of eligible and noneligible expenses to see whether specific mental health problems are included or excluded. Mental health benefits may be combined with medical benefits or they may be separate.

- What benefits do you get for mental health problems? Check the schedule of benefits carefully. The plan may set limits on payment for inpatient and outpatient treatment based on a certain number of days each year, a maximum cost per year, and/or a lifetime maximum.

- Are you required to use a certain provider? The insurance company may have a contract with a certain mental health center, thus limiting your options for selecting a provider.

- Who decides how much treatment you need? Some insurance companies look at your diagnosis and tell you how much treatment they will pay for. If your therapist thinks you need more, you may have to find the money for it yourself.

- Do the same rules apply? Your mental health benefits are probably subject to the same restrictions as your other benefits. For example, you may need to meet a yearly deductible before coverage begins, or you may need to get preauthorization.

- Will your employer find out if you use your mental health benefits? If your employer provides your health insurance, it may receive reports on who submits claims and for what. Your employer cannot release information about your claims to others and cannot use this information against you. Furthermore, most mental health professionals submit claims that maintain confidentiality.

My job offers a choice of health plans with different deductibles. How do I figure out which is best for me?

Here's how:

1. Using the deductible worksheet on p. 75, estimate constant costs (lines 1, 2, and 3). Start with yourself. What is the least amount you're likely to incur for covered health expenses in a year? Put that figure on line 1. Now, estimate the cost for your dependents who would be covered by the policy. Put those figures on lines 2 and 3.

2. Look at the deductibles for the policies you are thinking about (lines 4 and 10). Compare the deductibles to the constant costs for each member (lines 1, 2, and 3). Put the lowest number for each member on the appropriate line (lines 5, 6, and 7 for policy #1; lines 11, 12, and 13 for policy #2).

3. Write in the yearly cost of each policy (lines 8 and 14).

4. Calculate your yearly cost under each policy (lines 9 and 15).

5. Compare lines 9 and 15. The calculations you've done so far assume your family will have a healthy year. If the table shows that the policy with the higher deductible is cheaper overall, then you're done. This policy should be the cheapest for you every year. If instead the policy with the lower deductible is cheaper, which policy is best is less clear-cut. Fill out the table again. This time, instead of assuming everyone will need the least care possible, assume the expenses you actually expect.

Deductible Worksheet

	Family A	Family B	Your Family
Constant costs			
1. Member 1	$2,000	$2,000	_____
2. Member 2	$1,800	$400	_____
3. Member 3	$700	None	_____
Policy #1			
4. Deductible per person	$1,000	$1,000	_____
5. Unreimbursed costs for member 1: Put whichever is lower, line 1 or line 4	$1,000	$1,000	_____
6. Unreimbursed costs for member 2: Put whichever is lower, line 2 or line 4	$1,000	$400	_____
7. Unreimbursed costs for member 3: Put whichever is lower, line 3 or line 4	$700	$0	_____
8. Yearly policy cost	$4,000	$4,000	_____
9. Cost for year: Add lines 5–8	$6,700	$5,400	_____
Policy #2			
10. Deductible per person	$300	$300	_____
11. Unreimbursed costs for member 1: Put whichever is lower, line 1 or line 10	$300	$300	_____
12. Unreimbursed costs for member 2: Put whichever is lower, line 2 or line 10	$300	$300	_____
13. Unreimbursed costs for member 3: Put whichever is lower, line 3 or line 10	$300	$0	_____
14. Yearly policy cost	$5,000	$5,000	_____
15. Cost for year: Add lines 11–14	$5,900	$5,600	_____

Now that we have a son, my husband and I want to make sure he's cared for if something happens to us. How much life insurance do we need?

Congratulations on becoming parents! There's nothing like it in the world. You're right to want to take steps now to ensure that he is cared for financially. You may have heard rules of thumb for knowing how much life insurance you need—2 times your income, or 7 times your income. But it is far safer to work out the numbers for yourself. Here's how:

- Write down your current monthly after-tax income and expenses.
- Add up what your death will cost. Include the funeral and burial costs and the medical bills your health insurance won't cover. If you are wealthy, also include federal and state taxes.
- Estimate your family's monthly expenses after you die. One rule of thumb is that your family will need 75 percent of your after-tax income to keep up its standard of living.
- Estimate your family's monthly after-tax income. Include salaries, Social Security benefits, pensions, veterans' benefits, and any others.
- Figure the shortfall. Subtract what your family will need (step 3) from what it will take in (step 4). This is the monthly shortfall. If the amount is a negative number, multiply it by 12. This number is how much your family will fall short every year because of your absence (yearly shortfall). Then multiply that number by the number of years your family will need to be fed and clothed (lifetime shortfall).
- Calculate the total amount your family would need if you were to die. Take the lifetime shortfall you calculated in step 5 and add the death expenses from step 2. Are there other expenses you want to provide for? For example, you may want your family to have an emergency fund or be able to pay off debts. If so, add these expenses in as well.

- Finally, subtract any resources you have from what your family will need (step 6). For example, you may have savings accounts, individual retirement accounts, or investments. Or you may already have some life insurance.

After subtracting what you have from what your family will need, you have an approximate dollar number for the total amount of life insurance you need to buy.

・・・・・・・・・・・・・・・・・・・・・・・・・・・・・・・・・・・・・・・

I'm trying to find a life insurance company that accepts people with diabetes, and I'm getting nowhere. Can you help?

Because you have diabetes, obtaining life insurance may be harder than it is for other people. But don't despair. It's not impossible. There are companies willing to insure people with diabetes. Here are some ideas for tracking them down:

- See if your employer offers life insurance as part of your benefits package. Companies often have low group rates. You may not even need to answer any questions about your health.

- Check with your spouse's employer as well. At some companies, if an employee signs up for life insurance, the spouse can acquire a small add-on policy.

- Check with clubs, professional associations, college alumni associations, and trade groups. Some may offer life insurance at group rates. Consider joining a club or group just to buy life insurance. The club dues may be far less than the extra you'd have to pay for non-group insurance.

- If your life insurance needs are desperate, consider changing jobs for better life insurance. If you do so, make sure the terms of the insurance are in writing before making a move.

- If you can obtain only a small amount of life insurance from any one place, think about signing up anyway. You may be

INSURANCE 77

able to cobble together the coverage you need by having several tiny policies.

- Shop around. Just because one company turns you down doesn't mean they all will. Standards vary for deciding whether to insure someone. And some of those willing to insure you may "rate you up" more notches than others do.

- Look for "guaranteed acceptance" life insurance. Anybody can buy one of these policies. The catch: This insurance is very expensive, and you'll probably have to pay premiums for 2 or 3 years before full coverage kicks in.

I'm trying to decide between different kinds of life insurance. My agent wants me to get a "whole life" policy, but term insurance is a lot cheaper. What's your advice?

You are correct that term life insurance is cheaper; it is also the best choice for most people. Term insurance is like fire or car insurance: you buy a policy for a set amount of time, such as 5 years. Term rates do go up as you grow older. But your insurance needs usually go down as your children and your savings grow. Look for policies that are automatically renewable, have guaranteed premiums, and are convertible into cash-value insurance.

Cash-value insurance is more expensive than term insurance, but part of your fee earns tax-deferred interest. If you cancel the policy, you get money back. You can also take loans. And your premiums don't rise as you grow older. As with other investments, the "load" (administrative fees) you have to pay varies from policy to policy.

The two most common types of cash-value insurance are universal life and whole life. In whole life, your premiums are set. In universal life, you can vary how much and how often you pay. The insurance agent usually earns a commission from your first premiums, so you may not build up value in a cash-value policy for some time. On the other hand, some policies have no up-front sales fee when you buy, so it looks as if you're building value fast. But the policy may pay less interest, or you may have to pay a large fee if you cash in the policy early.

If you decide to go with a term policy, stick to your decision. Don't let the agent talk you into switching. Here are other term insurance tips:

- Look beyond the first year. Don't choose a term insurance policy based just on the first-year premium. Find out how often the premiums increase and whether there is a limit to how much they can go up.
- Choose a term policy that is renewable. Even though most people's insurance needs drop as they grow older, it's still a good idea to choose a policy that lets you convert to a cash-value policy—just in case you start a second family or your grandkids move in with you in your retirement years.
- Ignore most riders. Your family needs the same amount of money after you die whether you die in an accident or not.
- Study. Life insurance is very complex. You'll make a better decision if you read up on life insurance in consumer magazines and money-management books before shopping.

• •

 I've been offered a great new job. Trouble is, if I switch insurance, I'll have to worry about a preexisting-condition clause. What can you tell me about this?

 You are certainly warranted to be concerned about what kind of coverage you'll get at your next job. But you couldn't have picked a better time to want to change jobs. The Health Insurance Portability and Accountability Act of 1996 (effective 1 July 1997) makes it easier for people with diabetes to keep their health insurance when changing jobs.

According to the Act, if you have had diabetes for more than 6 months and have had continuous coverage in an insurance plan and then leave your job, you cannot be denied coverage by your new employer because of a preexisting condition.

If you have been recently diagnosed, that is, up to 6 months ago, and you change jobs, your new employer may refuse or limit your health insurance coverage for 12 months. But this is a one-time-only waiting period, and it can be reduced by the number of months you had continuous coverage at your previous job. For example, say you were diagnosed with diabetes while employed and covered by your employer's health insurance plan. Five months after the diagnosis, you change jobs. Your new employer may limit or deny your health insurance coverage for the remainder of the 12-month waiting period, or 7 months.

Another part of the Act states that all workers eligible for a particular health insurance plan must be offered enrollment at the same price. No more of this offering to cover you but only at a higher premium.

Get the full story about the company's health plan before accepting that new position. Try to obtain a dollars-and-cents answer to your coverage situation should you join the company. If the coverage will be more expensive than what you currently pay, try to negotiate that the difference be covered with a higher salary.

I've become disabled because of diabetes complications, and I want to apply for Social Security Disability. How do I do this?

For all the worried talk about Social Security's future, the program is alive and ready to help you. You can file for disability at your local Social Security office, or you can apply by phone or mail. (You will not receive any benefits for your first 6 months of disability.) If you go in person, take the following items:

- Your Social Security number
- Names, addresses, and phone numbers of providers and hospitals that have treated you
- The dates of treatment

- A list of the places you've worked in the past 15 years
- A summary of the work you've done in the past 15 years
- Proof of income (last year's W-2 if you worked for someone else or last year's federal tax form if you worked for yourself)

    The Social Security office first checks that you have enough credits in the right span of years. You earn credits based on how much money you made each year. How many credits and years you need depends on your age. For example, if you are 60, you need to have 40 credits, 20 of them earned within the past 10 years. But if you are 22, you need only 6 credits in the past 3 years.

    If you have enough credits, your application goes to your state's Disability Determination Services office. That office will decide whether you are disabled. It will collect reports from providers and institutions that have treated you. If that information is not enough, Social Security may pay for you to have a special exam.

    If you are approved, you can begin collecting benefits. If you are not approved, then you have 60 days to appeal the decision. Many disabled people have to appeal before being approved. Your monthly benefit depends on your lifetime average earnings. The more you earned, the higher your benefit will be. For more information, call Social Security on weekdays at 1-800-772-1213.

Chapter seven: CONSUMER ISSUES

Help! I just calculated this year's tax return and I owe a lot. What can I do as far as deducting medical expenses to cut my taxes next year?

Don't let the IRS get you down. With a little careful planning, you can greatly reduce the severity of next year's taxes.

First consider how many tax-deductible medical expenses you have collected for the year. You can deduct medical expenses only after the total exceeds 7.5 percent of your adjusted gross income.

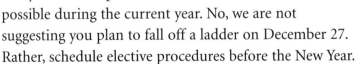

To lower your taxes, try to incur medical expenses in the year in which they'll help you the most. For instance, if you've already passed the 7.5 percent floor for the year, incur as many medical expenses as possible during the current year. No, we are not suggesting you plan to fall off a ladder on December 27. Rather, schedule elective procedures before the New Year.

On the other hand, if you expect to spend less than 7.5 percent of your income on medical bills, delaying some may let you deduct them next year. You can, for example, choose to hold off paying a medical bill that arrives in December but isn't due until January.

Another way to help yourself surpass the 7.5 percent floor is to schedule an elective surgery at the beginning of the year. This way you'll pay all the bills in one tax year instead of splitting costs over 2 years.

Another factor to include in your planning is next year's anticipated income. The higher your income, the higher your 7.5 percent floor. So it becomes harder to spend enough on medical bills to exceed it. Shifting expenses into the year in which you'll make less money, so that you can pass the floor, makes sense.

Enroll in a medical salary-reduction plan at work. If you have unreimbursed medical expenses every year, as most people with diabetes do, the plan allows you to pay those expenses with pre-tax income. Just be sure to use up all of the pre-tax income. If more money was taken from your pay than you paid in medical expenses, you lose the rest. Check where you stand in October and, if necessary, shift some medical expenses to the current year.

Diabetes costs a fortune. Sometimes I want to cut back on testing to save money. How can I save money but still take care of myself?

I know what you mean, and it's true, diabetes can be a budget-busting disease. But don't do something dangerous like not doing the tests you need. With a little budget tightening, you won't have to choose between safety and bankruptcy. Here are six ways to manage your medical costs:

1. Buy in bulk. You know you'll use up whatever diabetes supplies you buy, so it pays to stock up on items that are cheaper in large packages. Also, you can ask your doctor to write prescriptions for larger amounts. But be careful not to go over any quantity limits set by your insurance company for reimbursable items.

84 Dear Diabetes Advisor

2. Don't shoulder more than your share. Read your insurance policy with care to make sure you are not paying for covered items. Keep receipts so that you can prove your expenses.

3. Talk to your doctor about generic drugs. Generics are often cheaper and often work just as well. Both prescription and nonprescription drugs may be available as generics.

4. Look for house brand syringes. House brands are usually cheaper than name brands.

5. Talk to your doctor or nurse about reusing lancets and syringes. Although makers of syringes and lancets recommend that they be used only once, many health care providers believe that if you are careful, you can reuse them. Be sure to follow your health care provider's advice for cleaning and storing them.

6. Comparison shop. Before choosing a store, mail-order house, or club through which to buy your drugs, ask for a total price for all of them. (Don't bother asking about individual prices—it's best to keep all your prescriptions at the same place so that your pharmacist can warn you about interactions.) Also ask about discount plans for senior citizens or frequent buyers.

• •

My dietitian says, "Eat plenty of fresh fruits and vegetables." I say, "You come up with the money, then I'll eat healthy." How can I save on my grocery bills?

Let's get one thing straight. Eating healthy foods does not cost more. Fresh fruits, vegetables, grains, and legumes cost much less than meats and prepared foods. Perhaps it's other items you buy that are jacking up your grocery bills. Here are some ways to save:

- Compare the prices of the different stores in your area.
- Go to the store armed with a list, and stick to it. Don't give in to sudden impulse buying. It helps if you go shopping when you are not hungry.

CONSUMER ISSUES 85

- Don't buy special "diabetic" or "dietetic" foods. These are usually expensive. You can eat healthy with regular foods at regular prices.
- Clip coupons, keep them organized, and always take them with you when you go shopping. Shop on double-coupon days. Use coupons on sale items.
- Stock up on sale items that you use.
- Look for house brands. You'll save money and get nearly the same quality as name brands.
- Buy large or economy sizes; they're cheaper.
- If your store has a savings club, join it—it's usually free.
- Join a food co-op or club. You get near wholesale prices for buying foods in bulk (be sure you have someplace to store the huge quantities you have to buy).
- Keep track of what you are spending on food by deducting non-food items from your grocery bill. If you buy laundry detergent, shampoo, and other items at the supermarket, don't count them toward your food expenditures.
- Ask at the supermarket's fish department for fish scraps. They'll be free or very cheap. You can use them to make chowders and soups.
- Put family hunters and fishers to work. You can stock your freezer for the cost of a license.
- Grow your own vegetables and herbs in your backyard or on your windowsill or balcony.
- Look for "pick-your-own" farms and farmers' markets in your area. The cost is often lower. When they have too much, some farms will give away crops such as greens.

I receive a discount from my insurance company for ordering drugs by mail. Will I save money by using this service?

Not only will ordering your drugs by mail save you money, but your insurance company is going to give you a discount. Were you born lucky or what?

Mail-order services can buy large quantities of drugs and diabetes supplies at better prices. They can then offer you good discounts for more common drugs. For new or more expensive drugs, however, mail-order prices are close to the full price.

Do some comparison shopping of mail-order services before signing up. Most have toll-free 800 numbers for questions. Ask each mail-order service to give you the prices for the 1-month cost of all your drugs. Then compare the totals among all your "bidders."

Some mail-order services require customers to buy 3-month supplies. While this is a cost saver, just make sure it is within any limits set by your insurance company. And make sure your doctor understands how much you order so he or she can write your prescription for the proper amount.

One other thing to consider before you choose a mail-order service: Ask if you can use the toll-free 800 number to talk to a pharmacist—not just a salesperson—when you have problems or questions. A pharmacist's advice is especially helpful if you are trying new drugs or new nonprescription items.

Some mail-order services specialize in nonprescription items, such as blood glucose strips, monitors, and syringes. Explore these services, and you may be able to save even more money. To fill your order and arrange for insurance payment, most mail-order services need

- The original copy of your prescription mailed to them
- The information on your insurance card
- Time to fill the prescription (2 to 3 weeks)

CONSUMER ISSUES 87

Index

Acarbose, 8
Aging, 13, 57
Alpha-glucosidase inhibitors, 3
Anger, 39–41
Antioxidants, 43–44
Arthritis, 4, 30

Balloon angioplasty, 5–6
Biguanides, 3
Biofeedback, 34
Blood glucose, low, 16–17
Body mass index, 64
Bypass surgery, 5–6

Chocolate, 58–59
Cholesterol, 7
Chromium, 52
Coffee, 51–52

Dancing, 29–30
Deductible worksheet, 75
Dental care, 2
Depression, 37–38
Diabetes care, 11–13, 38–39
Diabetes pills, 3, 8
"Diabetes plus", 4–5
Dieting, 66–67
Disabled, 80–81

Exchanges, 47
Exercise, 21–32
   and fluids, 21–22
   minimum, 28–29
   pain, 22–23
   and travel, 31–32
Exercises
   aerobic, 22–23, 65–66
   dancing, 29–30
   flexibility, 25–27
   pool, 30–31
   strength, 27–28, 65–66
   stretching, 25–27
   walking, 23–24
   weight training, 27–28

Expenses
   grocery, 85–86
   medical, 83–85

Fast food, 55–56
Fat, 49–50
Flexibility, 25–27
Flu shot, 6
Fluids, 21–22
Food cravings, 58–59
Foods
   convenience, 52–53
   dietetic, 54–55
   snack, 59

Gallbladder, 1
Gallstones, 1
Grocery bills, 85–86
Gum disease, 2

Health care team, 11–12
Health Insurance Portability and
    Accountability Act of 1996, 79–80
Height and weight table, 64
Hypoglycemia, 16–17

Ice cream, 59
Impotence, 15
Insulin, 3
Insurance, 69–81
    health, 69–75, 79–81
    coverage
        for dietitian, 71
        for mental health, 72–73
        of preexisting condition, 79–80
    deductibles, 74–75
    life, 76–79
        finding, 77–78
        types of, 78–79
    terms, meaning of, 69–70

Mail order, 87
Managed care, 70–71
Marriage partner, 36–37
Medical expenses, 83–85
Medications, multiple, 3, 15–16
Minerals, 56–57
Mouth infections, 2

Neuropathy, 9–10
New Year's resolution, 35–36

Organized, getting, 38–39
Osteoporosis, 14, 56

Phytochemicals, 50–51
Preexisting condition, 79–80
Pregnancy, 18, 57
Prostate, 10–11

Relationships, 36–37

Salt, 48–49
Skin care, 19
Social Security Disability, 80–81
"Standards of Medical Care for Patients
    with Diabetes Mellitus," 11
Stress, 33–34
Stretching, 25–27
Sugar, 46
Sugar substitutes, 46
Sulfonylureas, 3

Taxes, 83–84
Teeth, 2
Telling others, 41–42
Thiazolidinediones, 3

Vegetarians, 44–45, 56

Walking, 23–24
Walking shoes, 24–25
Water, bottled, 57–58
Weight loss, 61–68
    diets, 66–67
    foods, 67–68
    goals, 63–65
    pills, 61–62
    programs, 62–63
Weight training, 27

Self-Care Titles

NEW!

Diabetes A to Z: What You Need to Know About Diabetes—Simply Put, 3rd Edition

This completely revised and updated guidebook is filled with the latest information on diabetes self care, including new medications, and treatment guidelines. You'll also learn all about blood sugar, complications, diet, exercise, and much more.

Softcover. #CGFDAZ
Nonmember: $11.95/ADA Member: $9.95

NEW!

Type 2 Diabetes: Your Healthy Living Guide, 2nd Edition

A thorough guide to staying healthy with type 2 diabetes—everything from choosing a health care team and eating and exercising to self-monitoring, insulin, and dealing with complications.

Softcover. #CTIIHG
Nonmember: $16.95/ADA Member: $14.95

NEW!

The Ten Keys to Helping Your Child Grow Up With Diabetes

A practical book for parents and caregivers of children with diabetes that addresses in detail the psychological, social, and emotional hurdles that often complicate the lives of youngsters with diabetes.

Softcover. #CSMTK
Nonmember: $14.95/ADA Member: $13.95

NEW!

Women & Diabetes

Designed for women, and filled with complete, thorough, and up-to-date discussions about a broad range of real-life topics such PMS, lactation, sex, pregnancy, child rearing, and menopause.

Softcover. #CSMWD
Nonmember: $14.95/ADA Member: $13.95

NEW!

Caring for the Diabetic Soul

You'll learn about coping with denial, controlling your stress and anger, building self-esteem, and much more. Written by professionals whose lives have been touched by diabetes—nurses, counselors, professors, doctors, and parents—each chapter reflects a personal experience that will touch you, too.

Softcover. #CSMCDS
Nonmember: $9.95/ADA Member: $8.95

NEW!

How to Get Great Diabetes Care

Informs you of the importance of seeking medical attention that meets the ADA Standards of Care.

Softcover. #CSMHGGDC
Nonmember: $11.95/ADA Member: $9.95

American Diabetes Association Complete Guide to Diabetes

Every area of self-care is covered in this ultimate diabetes reference for your home.
Hardcover. #CSMCGD
Nonmember: $29.95/ADA Member: $25.95

Paperback. #CSMCGDP (NEW!)
Nonmember: $19.95/ADA Member: $17.95

101 Tips for Staying Healthy with Diabetes

Get the inside track on the latest tips, techniques, and strategies for preventing and treating diabetes complications.

Softcover. #CSMFSH
Nonmember: $12.95/ADA Member: $10.95

Sweet Kids: How to Balance Diabetes Control & Good Nutrition with Family Peace

This new guide addresses behavioral and developmental issues of nutrition management.

Softcover. #CSMSK
Nonmember: $14.95/ADA Member: $11.95

Reflections on Diabetes

A collection of stories written by people who have learned from the experience of living with the disease.

Softcover. #CSMROD
Nonmember: $9.95/ADA Member: $8.95

101 Tips for Improving Your Blood Sugar

One question appears on each page, with the answers or "tips" below each question.

Softcover. #CSMTBBGC
Nonmember: $12.95/ADA Member: $10.95

Managing Diabetes on a Budget

For less than $10 you can begin saving hundreds and hundreds on your diabetes self-care.

Softcover. #CSMMDOAB
Nonmember: $7.95/ADA Member: $6.95

The Fitness Book: For People with Diabetes

You'll learn how to exercise to lose weight, exercise safely, get your mind and body ready to exercise, much more.

Softcover. #CSMFB
Nonmember: $18.95/ADA Member: $16.95

Raising a Child with Diabetes

Learn how to help your child adjust insulin to allow for foods kids like to eat, have a busy schedule, and much more.

Softcover. #CSMRACWD
Nonmember: $14.95/ADA Member: $12.95

The Dinosaur Tamer

Enjoy 25 fictional stories that will entertain, enlighten, and ease your child's frustrations about having diabetes.

Softcover. #CSMDTAOS
Nonmember: $9.95/ADA Member: $8.95

The Take-Charge Guide to Type I Diabetes

Discover how to prevent complications, learn all you can from testing your blood sugar, much more.

Softcover. #CSMT1
Nonmember: $16.95/ADA Member: $13.95

Diabetes & Pregnancy: What to Expect

You'll learn about an unborn baby's development, tests to expect, labor and delivery, birth control, much more.

Softcover. #CPREDP
Nonmember: $9.95/ADA Member: $8.95

Gestational Diabetes: What to Expect

Discover what gestational diabetes is and how to care for yourself during your pregnancy.

Softcover. #CPREGD
Nonmember: $9.95/ADA Member: $8.95

Necessary Toughness

You'll be inspired by this story of an athlete with the courage to face not only NFL linemen but also the threat of diabetes.

Softcover. #CGFNT
Nonmember: $7.95/ADA Member: $6.95

Diabetes: A Positive Approach—Video

#CVIDPOS
Nonmember: $19.95/ADA Member: $17.95

1998 Buyer's Guide

#CMISBUY98
Nonmember: $4.95/ADA Member: $3.95

Cookbooks & Meal Planners

NEW!

The Diabetes Carbohydrate and Fat Gram Guide

Registered dietitian Lea Ann Holzmeister shows you how to count carbohydrate and fat grams and exchanges, and why it's important. Dozens of charts list foods, serving sizes, and nutrient data for hundreds of products.

Softcover. #CMPCFGG
Nonmember: $11.95/ADA Member: $9.95

NEW!

Brand-Name Diabetic Meals

Save time cooking with these popular taste-tested recipes from the kitchens of Campbell Soup, Kraft Foods, Weetabix, Dean Foods, Eskimo Pie, and Equal. Features more than 200 recipes from appetizers to desserts.

Softcover. #CCBBNDM
Nonmember: $12.95/ADA Member: $10.95

NEW!

How to Cook for People with Diabetes

Finally, a collection of reader favorites from the delicious, nutritious recipes featured every month in *Diabetes Forecast*.

Softcover. #CCBCFPD
Nonmember: $11.95/ADA Member: $9.95

NEW!

Magic Menus

Now you can plan all your meals from more than 50 breakfasts, 50 lunches, 75 dinners, and 30 snacks. Like magic, this book figures fats, calories, and exchanges for you automatically. The day's calories will still equal 1,500.

Softcover. #CCBMM
Nonmember: $14.95/ADA Member: $12.95

Diabetic Meals In 30 Minutes—Or Less!

Put an end to bland, time-consuming meals with more than 140 fast, flavorful recipes. Complete nutrition information accompanies every recipe. Includes a number of "quick tips."

Softcover. #CCBDM
Nonmember: $11.95/ADA Member: $9.95

Diabetes Meal Planning Made Easy

Understand how to use the Nutrition Facts on food labels. You'll also master the new Diabetes Food Pyramid.

Softcover. #CCBMP
Nonmember: $14.95/ADA Member: $12.95

Month of Meals

When celebrations begin, go ahead—dig in! Enjoy Chicken Cacciatore, Oven Fried Fish, Sloppy Joes, and many others.

Softcover. #CMPMOM
Nonmember: $12.50/ADA Member: $10.50

Month of Meals 2

Automatic menu planning goes ethnic! Tips and meal suggestions for your favorite restaurants are featured.

Softcover. #CMPMOM2
Nonmember: $12.50/ADA Member: $10.50

Month of Meals 3

Enjoy fast food without guilt! Make delicious choices at McDonald's, Wendy's, and other fast food restaurants.

Softcover. #CMPMOM3
Nonmember: $12.50/ADA Member: $10.50

Month of Meals 4

Meat and potatoes menu planning! Enjoy with old-time family favorites like Meatloaf and Pot Roast.

Softcover. #CMPMOM4
Nonmember: $12.50/ADA Member: $10.50

Month of Meals 5

Meatless meals picked fresh from the garden. Choose from a garden of fresh vegetarian selections.

Softcover. #CMPMOM5
Nonmember: $12.50/ADA Member: $10.50

To order call 1-800-232-6733 and mention code CK897DDA.

To join ADA call: 1-800-806-7801

About the American Diabetes Association

The American Diabetes Association is the nation's leading voluntary health organization supporting diabetes research, information, and advocacy. Founded in 1940, the Association supports an office in every state and provides services to communities across the country. Its mission is to prevent and cure diabetes and to improve the lives of all people affected by diabetes.

For more than 50 years, the American Diabetes Association has been the leading publisher of comprehensive diabetes information for people with diabetes and the health care professionals who treat them. Its huge library of practical and authoritative books for people with diabetes covers every aspect of self-care—cooking and nutrition, fitness, weight control, medications, complications, emotional issues, and general self-care. The Association also publishes books and medical treatment guides for physicians and other health care professionals.

Membership in the Association is available to health care professionals and people with diabetes and includes subscriptions to one or more of the Association's periodicals. People with diabetes receive *Diabetes Forecast*, the nation's leading health and wellness magazine for people with diabetes. Health care professionals receive one or more of the Association's five scientific and medical journals.

For more information, please call toll-free

Questions about diabetes:	1-800-DIABETES
Membership, people with diabetes:	1-800-806-7801
Membership, health professionals:	1-800-232-3472
Free catalog of ADA books:	1-800-232-6733
Visit us on the Web:	www.diabetes.org
Visit us at our Web bookstore:	www.diabetes.store